DARE TO DETOX

AN INTEGRATIVE APPROACH TO RENEWING YOUR BODY, MIND AND SPIRIT

GRETCHEN REIS, MD

DISCLAIMER

This book is not intended as a substitute for the medical advice of a physician. The reader should regularly consult a physician in matters relating to his or her health and particularly with respect to any symptoms that may require diagnosis or medical attention. Statements regarding products have not been evaluated by the Food and Drug Administration. Any products or treatment regimens are not intended to diagnose, treat, cure or prevent any disease. If you are pregnant, nursing, taking medication, or have a medical condition, consult your health care professional before using any products based on this content. The information in this book is for general health knowledge only. Results of medical treatments vary and the author assumes no liability or responsibility for any actions taken by the reader or any outcomes thereof.

"One of the most confusing issues for patients is detoxification. Dr. Reis gives us a wonderfully easy and thorough answer to that confusion in this guide. From what toxins are and their effects on our bodies, to how to detox your life for both physical and mental health, this is an amazing guide."

— BENITA PHILLIPS DO, ALIVE AND WELL HEALTH

"Dr. Reis has provided an easy to understand, quick read that provides a complete look into the how-tos of detox. This is a great resource for patients and doctors alike."

— JULIA KISSEL MD, RESTORATIVE WELLNESS MD

"Dr. Reis gives a great concise yet thorough account of what we integrative doctors want our patients to know about detoxification. This easy-to-read guide will serve as a primer for my patients. They will further enjoy knowing she has helped thousands of patients restore their health through a holistic, comprehensive approach."

— BRYAN WARNER MD, HEALTH BY DESIGN MD

DEDICATION

To my colleagues in integrative medicine, who constantly inspire me to do more to help my patients reach their health goals,

To my staff for their encouragement to write this book,

And to my husband Bill, for his tireless encouragement in the ministry of holistic health.

CONTENTS

INTRODUCTION

Toxins, detox, cleanse, flush. You've probably heard all these terms but perhaps haven't quite understood exactly what they mean. Do toxins really affect our health? What is a detox? Pills and powders? Eating only plants or just drinking juice for a month? Who really needs to do a detox? What is the best one to do?

These are all very good questions that unfortunately, are often not addressed by the medical community. There are a lot of misconceptions out there about how toxins affect our bodies and metabolism, as well as what works to reduce their effect. Physicians often will tell you that there is no reason to do a detox, but that is simply because there is no consensus on which of the many types of detox programs marketed actually are useful. There are also a lot of different definitions for the term "detox", which creates significant confusion among patients and physicians. Also, most physicians are hesitant to recommend anything that isn't based on a peer-reviewed clinical study. Lastly, many physicians simply have not taken the time to learn about detoxification strategies, which are simply enhancing the natural detoxification processes the body uses, so they avoid recommending anything at all.

Before we talk about detoxification itself, let's go on a journey first to explore toxins and what they can do to us. Hold on tight: it's pretty terrifying.

TOXINS: WHERE ARE THEY?

*T*oxins are everywhere, both in our environment and in our cells. First of all, keep in mind that normally, our cells produce some natural byproducts of cellular metabolism that can be considered cellular toxins. The natural process of cellular detoxification normally works well. One example is an enzyme that turns a toxin into something harmless, and then it is recycled or eliminated. But in some chronic diseases, this natural cleansing mechanism is sluggish. Cells may not have the right nutrients or energy needed to accomplish these reactions. Toxins in the cells then build up. Add to that a significant exposure to toxins from the outside world, and then the body is less able to detoxify even natural cellular waste. Unless the overall toxin load comes down, the cells and the body will struggle to perform as they are designed to do. Ultimately, we feel the effects.

Toxins are everywhere in our environment.[1] Some toxins are obvious, like fumes when filling up the gas tank, but some are not so obvious, like the phthalates in that scented candle that smells so nice. Dryer sheets, household cleaners, pesticides, and new construction materials can put toxins in our homes. Food cans, drinking water, meat and produce have toxins. Many personal care products like body wash, nail polish and perfume or cologne have toxins. That list doesn't even count what's in the garage or the basement! Add to that the air we breathe and I promise that we are exposed to many more toxins than we are aware of. This is just the world we live in now. Compared to only 100 years ago, our environment is completely different and it is often making us sick.

We eat toxins in our food, we breathe toxins in our air, and we absorb toxins through our skin every day. There have been over 80,000 chemicals registered for use in the United States according to the US Department of Health and Human Services.[2] Over 2000 new chemicals are registered every year! They end up in our food, personal care products, lawn care products and in our air. We are awash in chemicals.

Do toxins really get into our bodies? The answer is a resounding yes! In 2009 the Centers for Disease Control released their "Fourth Report on Human Exposure to Environmental Chemicals".[3] This showed that **hundreds** of chemicals are present in most people. Other studies have shown phthalates (from plastic) were present in 75% of the population, and bisphenol A (BPA) was found in 95% of people! [4,5]

The Environmental Working Group did a landmark study of newborns in 2004 that had absolutely shocking results.[6] These newborns had their umbilical cord blood tested for 287 different toxins, including PCB's, dioxin, flame retardants, DDT, pesticides and mercury. **Every one of them** tested positive and the average number of toxins present was over 200!

So if children are born already polluted, how do you think we are doing as adults? It's a sobering thought.

Mainstream medicine often sticks its head in the sand at this point. Evidence continues to accumulate that these toxins are in many of our bodies, and new links between certain toxins and chronic disease are being discovered all the time. But physicians commonly believe that in the low doses most of us are exposed to, these chemicals don't harm humans. While that is true to some degree, often it is not. Small doses here and there in someone who is otherwise healthy and has a strong detoxification system will not generally cause symptoms.

But what if someone cannot detoxify well? Genetics, inflammation, disease, nutrient deficiencies and medications all can decrease detoxification ability. Also, if a person has multiple toxins in their system at the same time, their detoxification pathways can be overwhelmed.

Let's take a look at some of the most common toxins in our environment and what they can do to us.

COMMON TOXINS

- **Bisphenol-A (BPA)**

Found in plastics, thermal receipts, bottled water, soda cans and food cans. BPA can disrupt thyroid and sex hormones and can cause macrosomia (large birth weight babies). In utero exposure can cause polycystic ovarian syndrome (PCOS) to emerge years later which is a leading cause of infertility. BPA is also linked to cancer, diabetes, heart disease, and obesity.[7, 8, 9, 10]

- **Phthalates**

Found in detergents, cosmetics (especially nail polish), plastics, soap, paint and perfume. "Fragrance" usually is diethyl phthalate so avoid air fresheners, scented candles and perfume. It also is found in insect repellants, adhesives, and varnishes. Phthalates disrupt hormones, cause diabetes, promote cancer, cause asthma, affect sexual development of children and lead to obesity.[11] There is also a "phthalate syndrome"[12] described in men, which is low sperm counts, infertility, obesity and diabetes. One study found phthalates in over 93% of pregnant women's urine.[13]

- **Parabens**

Preservatives found in body wash, shampoo and lotions. They are associated with breast cancer and disrupt hormones.[14]

- **Polybrominated diphenylethers (PBDE's)**

Found in flame retardants, furniture foam, plastics in appliances and electronics. There is some evidence that PBDE's may be associated with thyroid hormone disruption or perhaps even thyroid cancer.[15]

- **Polychlorinated biphenyls (PCB's)**

Environmental chemicals not made in the US for decades, but persist long-term in the environment. Exposure to PCB's is typically from food or air. PCB's are present in grass, so even grass fed beef can have PCB's, as can organic butter. They disrupt hormonal systems, can increase the risk of certain cancers, and may be linked to dementia and Parkinson's disease.[16, 17, 18]

- **PVC**

Used to make inexpensive children's toys (plastic books or toys), shower curtains, and vinyl flooring. PVC releases unhealthy fumes into the air, such as formaldehyde. It often also contains phthalates and lead. It can affect the nervous system, liver and bone health.[19]

- **Atrazine**

An herbicide used on corn crops and found in drinking water. It is associated with hormone disruption in animals and may do the same in humans.[20] There is also some concern that it may increase risk for ovarian cancer.[21]

- **Triclosan**

An antibacterial agent added to soaps. Triclosan causes liver scarring and tumors in rodents. In humans, it can affect the thyroid or cause allergies.[22, 23, 24]

- **Pesticides**

Organophosphates, the most common type of pesticide, may be linked to developmental delay, autism spectrum disorder and preterm labor in pregnant women.[25, 26] They are neurotoxic acutely, so chronic low level exposure is not healthy for neurologic function. Estimates are that over 60% of American children have pesticides in their urine! They also may affect the immune system, may increase cancer risk and are linked to asthma.[27, 28]

- **Herbicides (glyphosate)**

Roundup™, the most commonly used weed killer, contains glyphosate and other ingredients that are toxic. This product was at the center of a number of lawsuits that Bayer recently settled without acknowledging any connection between its product and disease.[29] However, many in the medical community, in particular environmental medicine experts, are very concerned about all herbicides, especially glyphosate. Glyphosate has been associated with death of testicular cells and is commonly found in men who have low testosterone and erectile dysfunction in their thirties and forties[30]. It can also disrupt hormones in women.[31] Other possible consequences of herbicide exposure may be obesity, diabetes, hypertension and dementia. Herbicides have been associated with cancer, kidney disease, asthma, and neurologic issues including seizures.[32]

- **Vehicle exhaust**

Exhaust contains MTBE and ETBE, which are gasoline additives. Commuters in larger cities are often exposed to significant vehicle exhaust. MTBE and ETBE are also commonly found in groundwater supplies. These chemicals can damage the liver, kidneys, nervous system and may promote cancer.[33, 34]

- **Volatile organic compounds (VOC's)**

Found in paint, varnish, new carpeting, building materials, and household cleaners. VOC's can cause asthma, headaches and can suppress cellular metabolism.[35, 36]

- **Perchloroethylene**

Used in dry cleaning solvents, associated with cancer.[37]

- **Xylene**

Found in paint, pesticides, fuel fumes, perfume and insect repellants. High levels can cause dizziness, headaches, incoordination, shortness of breath and chest pain.[38]

- **Styrene**

Used in food packaging (styrofoam), building materials and vehicle exhaust. It is an irritant and can affect the nervous system as well as increasing the risk for leukemia, lymphoma and a type of nasal cancer.[39, 40]

- **Perfluorooctanoic acid (PFOA)**

Used in non-stick cookware, in carpeting and in the lining of popcorn bags. It is associated with testicular and kidney cancer, increased cholesterol and thyroid disorders.[41]

- **Benzene**

Solvent that is widespread; comes from industrial processes, vehicle exhaust and cigarette smoke. It can cause nausea, cognitive impairment, and dizziness. Benzene damages DNA and can cause leukemia.[42]

- **Acrylamide**

Formed when starchy foods are heated in oil (i.e. fried) at high temperatures (like French fries and potato chips). Acrylamide is also present in plastics, some cosmetics, and cigarette smoke. It causes neurologic damage, decreased reproduction and cancer in animals.[43, 44]

- **Heavy metals**

Lead is found in water pipes, lipstick and some hair dyes. Mercury is in dental amalgams ("silver" fillings) and fish. Cadmium is prevalent in cigarette smoke. Arsenic can be found in small amounts in rice, chicken and even in the municipal water supply. Mercury has been linked to autoimmune diseases and neurological symptoms.[45, 46] This is characterized by the expression "mad as a hatter", which was from the mercury used in hatmaking in the 19th century. Arsenic is associated with lung, skin and bladder cancer.[47] Lead toxicity in children is associated with developmental delay.[48] Cadmium is well known to affect the kidneys and increases the risk of osteoporosis.[49, 50]

- **Acrolein**

Herbicide used in stagnant water to kill algae. It also is found in food, water, cigarette smoke and vehicle exhaust. Acrolein may be a factor in cardiovascular disease.[51]

- **Perchlorate**

Perchlorate is often found in produce and milk, as well as fertilizers, fireworks, rocket fuel and bleach. It competes with iodine for a place in thyroid hormone synthesis, affecting thyroid hormone levels.[52]

- **Plastics**

Plastic containers have a variety of chemical compounds. Every plastic container has a recycling symbol with a number, ranging from 1 to 7, within a triangle. Since there are such a wide variety of plastic types, and some are definitely worse for you than others, here is a list of the codes.

Remember, though, no matter what: NEVER microwave in plastic! All you are doing is driving the chemical directly into your food or beverage. I also caution you to avoid making a habit of drinking coffee brewed in individual plastic pods. The hot coffee drips through a puncture in the plastic. Depending on which plastic type it is and how often you drink it, that may add up to significant toxin exposure.

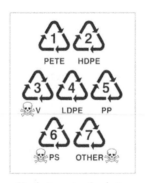

Numbering system for plastics

1. PETE or PET (polyethylene terephthalate)

Found mostly in packaging for soda, water, peanut butter, mouthwash, and salad dressing

2. HDPE (high density polyethylene)

Containers for milk, juice, water, margarine, detergent and cleaners

3. PVC/vinyl

Shampoo bottles, cooking oil bottles, food shrink wrap, and windows

4. LDPE (low density polyethylene)

Shopping bags, squeezable bottles, milk jugs, bread bags, some food wrap

5. PP (polypropylene)

Ketchup and syrup bottles, yogurt containers, margarine tubs

6. PS (polystyrene)

Foam food trays, coffee cup lids (you may not have ever thought of this one, but don't drink hot coffee through a plastic lid!), egg cartons and Styrofoam plates and cups

7. Other (BPA, polycarbonate, others)

Cans, baby bottles, large water bottles, some food packaging.

Most Toxic	Least Toxic
3	2
6	4
7	5

Effects of toxins

With this frightening list of toxins in our world, there is a lot that can go wrong medically. Since cancer is certainly one of the more serious conditions we fear, let's start here.

Cancers of virtually all types have been associated with different toxins. Liver cancer is a well-known cancer that can be a result of alcoholism. Lung cancer certainly occurs much more often in smokers, as well as bladder cancer being more common in smokers.[53] But there are a lot of other kinds of cancer, such as brain, stomach, kidney, breast, colon, prostate and others. Some of them are related to toxins.

The problem here is that toxins damage DNA in a cell, which essentially short-wires the cell, and it can become cancerous. If the immune system isn't up to the challenge of killing the first few early cancer cells, the cancer spreads and then overcomes the immune system. It then takes heavy doses of toxic chemotherapy or radiation to kill the cancer cells.

Toxic effects of chemicals can include:

- Allergies and asthma
- Immune disorders
- Diabetes
- Hormone imbalance
- Infertility
- Brain dysfunction
- Birth defects
- Autism spectrum disorders and developmental delay
- ADHD
- Anxiety and depression
- Birth defects

- Cancer
- Neurologic diseases

Neurologic problems are very common as well. There are concerns that toxins can contribute to Parkinson's disease, Alzheimer's, ALS, and multiple sclerosis. Many people with acute toxin exposure initially have dizziness, headaches, and cognitive slowing (brain fog). It isn't a stretch to imagine that chronic exposure can affect the cells of the nervous system, especially the brain, and cause disease.

The entire endocrine system is also highly susceptible to toxins: blood sugar regulation (diabetes), thyroid hormone, and sex hormones all can be significantly affected and cause disease. As a physician specializing in bioidentical hormones, it is stunning how often we see men and women with hormonal issues at much younger ages than we used to see a few decades ago. Premenstrual syndrome (PMS), polycystic ovarian syndrome (PCOS), and endometriosis have become quite common in women. One way this can happen is a condition called estrogen dominance.

Normally, estrogen and progesterone fluctuate through the monthly cycle in a well-defined way. Overall, their effects are balanced one to another. However, many toxins are "xenoestrogens", which means they activate the estrogen receptors.[54] They have a chemical structure that is in some way similar enough to estrogen, so that they can latch onto an estrogen receptor and activate the cell. This causes a dominance of estrogen effect, called estrogen dominance. When estrogen effect dominates over progesterone effect, the result can be heavy periods or PMS.[55]

In men, toxins can do two things. First, they can damage the pituitary gland or the testes, so the body simply doesn't make enough testosterone. Testosterone deficiency causes low libido, fatigue, low motivation, ED, and less muscle mass. Secondly, toxins can be xenoestrogens. Even if your testosterone level is normal, the activation of estrogen receptors can blunt the natural effect of testosterone, so you feel like your testosterone level is low.

How common is this? More common than most realize. Have you noticed the advertisements for the telemedicine companies selling ED (erectile dysfunction) medication? Why are men in their 30's and 40's needing medication for ED? Why are physicians like me seeing more men under 50 needing testosterone therapy to regain their health? Are you connecting the dots yet?

I recently saw a 38 year old man who came in for low libido, brain fog, weight gain, depression and low motivation. His testosterone level, which should be 500-1200, was only 137! When I took a detailed history, I discovered that he bought a lawn care business when he was 21, and he worked it by himself for about 10 years before he sold the business. All that time he was spraying herbicides on a daily basis. He was no longer in exposure, but all that exposure severely damaged his testicular cells. As a result, he is now on testosterone therapy, which he will need the rest of his life. He now lives a lower toxin lifestyle but he wishes he had known about this when he was 21.

Birth defects are clearly caused by toxins of all sorts.[56] Fetal alcohol syndrome is fairly common, but obviously, drugs of all sorts can wreak havoc on a baby in utero. For the most part, we all know not to drink alcohol, smoke cigarettes or do other drugs when pregnant, but it's the small exposures we are completely unaware of that can do severe damage.

So what do we physicians see in our patients? We have discussed hormone imbalance. Toxins clearly are a leading cause of low testosterone in men and infertility in women.[57, 58] Diabetes and obesity, often called "diabesity", is widespread in our nation. We have evidence that BPA and phthalates can increase the risk of diabetes.[59, 60] There are also numerous studies linking various cancers to different toxins. Lastly, toxins are associated with allergies, autism and ADHD.[61, 62, 63] Geographical data have shown an interesting correlation. When looking at a map of the USA showing the prevalence of autism spectrum disorders, it is quite similar to maps showing the prevalence of toxins in the environment.[64, 65] Could one reason for the steady increase in autism be environmental toxins? Many physicians say yes.

One of the most common medical issues that is related to toxin exposure is absolutely everywhere: obesity. The rates of obesity have skyrocketed in the US over the past 30 years. What used to be only a mild problem is now ubiquitous. Around two-thirds of Americans are overweight, and around 40% are clinically obese.[66] Have you ever really thought about why that is?

Certainly, the advancements in technology have caused a shift in the workplace from manual labor to more sedentary jobs, but it's not just that. Food choices are also certainly to blame. With the misguided emphasis on low-fat diets in the past few decades, Americans shifted to eating more carbohydrates. This did not solve the problem, however, and in fact likely worsened it. Obesity rates continued to rise. The proliferation of fast food and high sugar, nutrient-poor convenience foods have made it much easier to consume a lot of sugar in a short time. All these things make it much harder to keep a healthy weight, especially with aging.

If you start to look at toxins in our food supply, however, you will find a deeply concerning trend. Grains, legumes, fruits and vegetables grown in the US are more and more often incorporating toxins from the soil, air, and the water. Glyphosate is found in the soil and water far away from where it is actually applied to the land.[67] Pesticides, heavy metals and other industrial chemicals get into the water supply and even into the air.

They get into the food being grown, and then we eat it. Many toxins affect the insulin sensitivity of cells, which means your blood sugar levels stay higher after eating. Insulin causes fat storage, so too much for too long causes weight gain.

Toxins may also affect leptin receptors. Leptin is a hormone that is supposed to burn calories and drive cellular metabolism. But sometimes people get leptin resistance, which is one reason why losing weight seems nearly impossible. So toxins really might be a reason why some people just cannot lose weight, even with a healthy low carbohydrate diet and moderate exercise.

Be aware, though, that toxins do not always produce overt disease or even weight gain. They can be very sneaky. Many people are overall fairly healthy, but they just don't feel well sometimes. They may feel tired, bloated or have headaches. Maybe it's joint pain or muscle pain. Sometimes it's mood swings or trouble focusing. These seemingly minor symptoms may not be enough for a formal medical diagnosis, but they all can be related to some level of toxin exposure. That's because the toxins accumulate and suppress how well cells and bodily systems function. If your heart works pretty well but not great, you may get short of breath with a lesser amount of exercise or you may get palpitations. Perhaps your digestion will be off in a mild way causing bloating or diarrhea. Women may have irregular periods. Men and women alike can have trouble with sexual health. If the brain isn't optimally healthy, moods can fluctuate and significant brain fog may occur.

This is where it gets challenging. Many of these symptoms are quite normal in most of us at certain times! No one feels great all the time. So what level of symptoms is normal? It is hard to say. However, if people have significant toxin exposure and aren't even looking for these patterns, they can be missed.

Healthcare practitioners often simply prescribe medication for individual symptoms. For example, if you see a gastroenterologist for bloating and abdominal pain, you will be probably diagnosed with irritable bowel syndrome and be given a prescription for the pain. The doctor most likely won't mention eliminating gluten and dairy or ask you about toxin exposure. Unfortunately, most physicians simply have no time during a regular office visit to do this. Prescribing medications is what they are trained to do, but totally misses the underlying cause. It's up to you to try to decode the signals your body is giving you and to do all you can to create the right environment for your body to heal. Now we can talk about detoxification!

NATURAL DETOXIFICATION PROCESSES

hen we ingest or absorb toxins, we depend on our body to eliminate them promptly. There are 5 main pathways our bodies use to rid ourselves of toxic substances:

1. Liver
2. Kidney
3. Gut
4. Skin
5. Lungs

Our bodies are actually very good at this. Whenever there are redundant systems in the body, if one gets sluggish, the others can ramp up to compensate. But over time, if toxins accumulate and cellular metabolism is affected, detoxification ability gets slower, compounding the problem. Keep in mind that when we talk about a "detox program", all we really are talking about is creating an environment that optimizes our body's own naturally occurring detoxifying processes. We are enhancing **what our bodies naturally do.**

The liver often gets the most attention, because it is crucial for detoxification. There are two phases to detoxification in the liver, called Phase 1 and Phase 2. There is also a so-called Phase 3 detoxification pathway, which is the bile going into the colon and then wastes going out in bowel movements, but for now, let's talk about Phases 1 and 2 that occur in the liver.

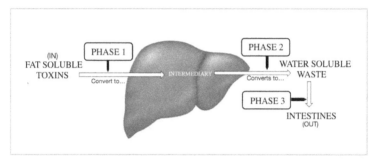

Liver detoxification

Phase 1

Phase 1 is where the liver takes the toxin and actually converts it to a highly reactive metabolite. This involves a group of enzymes called the cytochrome P450 family. This would not be good if the process stopped there, because these metabolites can damage proteins and DNA. The most recognized process of all these is oxidation, where oxygen reacts with a substance to produce a more unstable substance. The best-known example of oxidation is when oxygen reacts with iron to cause rust. However, other mechanisms are listed in the box below. Phase 1 reactions are dependent on a number of B vitamins as well as glutathione and flavonoids. The end result of Phase 1 is an unstable molecule that can actually damage cells. But thankfully, the process doesn't end there; it goes on to Phase 2.

Phase 1
(Cytochrome P450 Enzymes)
Oxidation
Reduction
Hydrolysis
Hydration
Dehalogenation

Nutrients Needed
Vitamins B2, B3, B6, B12
Folate
Glutathione
Flavonoids

Phase 2

Phase 2 is attaching a molecule to that toxic metabolite to neutralize it, and to prepare it for elimination. There are 6 ways the liver can accomplish this: acetylation, amino acid conjugation, glucuronidation, conjugation to glutathione, methylation and sulfation.

Once these things are conjugated, or attached, to the toxin, it is stable and can be eliminated in the stool or urine. The liver needs certain nutrients to accomplish this conjugation: amino acids, glutathione, sulfur and certain B vitamins. This is why we supplement amino acids and B vitamins during detoxification.

PHASE 2: (CONJUGATION PATHWAYS)

Phase 2
(Conjugation Pathways)
Acetylation
Amino acid conjugation
Glucuronidation
Glutathione conjugation
Methylation
Sulfation

Nutrients Needed
Methionine
Cysteine
Magnesium
Glutathione
Pantothenic Acid
Vitamin B12
Vitamin C
Glycine
Taurine
Glutamine
Folate
Choline

The kidneys also eliminate toxins in the urine. This is one reason why drinking plenty of water is good for you. This is a powerful pathway for detoxification for many substances, so maintaining a healthy blood pressure is important for good kidney function.

The intestines are also very important. After Phase 2 conjugation, the liver excretes toxins into the bile which gets dumped into the small intestine. However, if the gut is sluggish and one is constipated, the toxins will not be eliminated like they should. Some of them can be reabsorbed as they travel down the intestine, which is the exact opposite of what we want. This is one reason why a healthy gut is so important. Good things (nutrients) are supposed to get absorbed, but bad things (toxins, inflammatory foods) are supposed to be eliminated. A major strategy of a good detoxification regimen is eliminating foods that commonly cause gut inflammation: gluten, dairy, and corn are a few examples. Eating healthy, whole foods that are anti-inflammatory will enhance intestinal health, which helps the toxins travel all the way through the gut and out.

Don't forget about our skin and lungs...they also help with detoxification. Exercise can generate a good sweat, which helps rid the body of toxins. Saunas and sweating can be helpful. The lungs have a role to play, also. Have you ever eaten a keto diet and had "ketone breath"? When diabetics get into ketoacidosis (from very high blood sugar levels), they have ketone breath. The body breathes off excess ketones in the lungs. One more reason not to smoke is to preserve your lungs' ability to eliminate toxins.

But if we are exposed to more toxins than our livers can handle, the toxins will be stored in our bodies. For example, if you drink alcohol every day, your liver is busy detoxifying that and it then cannot process other environmental toxins. The biggest storage place for toxins is fat cells.[68] These stored toxins can affect the body in many ways for a long time, and it is difficult to eliminate them.

This is a good time to note that genetics play a big role in detoxification. There are genetic tests we can do to assess certain enzymes in the body that affect detoxification. For example, glutathione S-transferase (GST) and methylenetetrahydrofolate reductase (MTHFR) are two enzymes important in Phase 2 liver detoxification. Some of us have genetic variants that make these enzymes less effective than normal. This likely is a reason why some people live around high levels of toxins but never get sick (like the smoker who lives until age 90 and never gets cancer) or why some people get sick quite easily when young.

This is why you cannot assume one person has the same detoxification ability as the next person! There is a lot of individual variation.

If functional genetic testing is done and genetic enzyme weaknesses are found, extra nutrients can be taken which help support those enzymes. Ask your provider for information on this testing.

DETOXIFICATION IN HISTORY AND NOW

*D*etoxification is not new! Cultures and societies have incorporated types of detoxification practices for centuries. Biblical societies and religious cultures of old often implemented periods of fasting. Fasting is completely depriving your body of incoming nutrients and resting the bowel. While this is difficult and often unnecessary, it does allow the body to detoxify.

The Jewish faith has practiced fasting for thousands of years. Islam and then Christianity have incorporated fasting as well. Muslims fast during the day for Ramadan and Christians often set aside time to pray and fast. There is often great value in changing your daily routine away from eating and focusing on spiritual activities. Millions of people have experienced the spiritual and physical cleansing benefits from this practice. Well known scriptures include:

I humbled myself with fasting.

— PSALM 35:13

...this kind (of spiritual difficulty) does not go out except by prayer and fasting.

— MATTHEW 17:21

When preparing to detox, keep in mind that mental health and spiritual health go hand in hand with physical detoxification. In fact, here is something to ponder:

If your body is detoxed and healthy but your mind or your soul is troubled and unwell, have you really accomplished anything?

More on this later, but for now, I encourage you to consider how you can "detox" your mind, your thoughts, and your soul. Take some time to detoxify your mind from useless television and social media. Turn off the news. Limit the use of electronics or video games. Read a book on self-improvement. Seek God and His purpose for your life. Be a blessing to others. Learn how to be less selfish and give more. Release anger and resentment you may be harboring and forgive. There is nothing more powerful spiritually than forgiving others and receiving forgiveness. Detoxify hate and anger; receive healing and peace in your heart. It can truly transform your life!

This is a personal and unique journey for each of us, but please do not simply focus on what you can and cannot eat and what supplements to take. Broaden your vision and approach this holistically. We are body, mind and soul. Don't ignore those other parts.

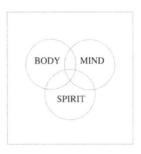

Detoxification has become very popular, and there are a lot of different types of "cleanses" out there. Some of them are "liver cleanses", and some are bowel cleanses. The latter typically include high doses of laxatives or even colonic irrigation, which is a temporary cleansing of the intestines. While most people do feel less bloated after the intestines are cleared, it is only short-lived and sometimes unsafe. Electrolyte imbalances can occur which can cause cardiac rhythm issues and dehydration. This is not truly a whole body detox regimen.

Other cleanses involve diuretics, or water pills. These will definitely increase urination, but again, this can cause dehydration or electrolyte imbalances. This is not truly a detox.

Lastly, some people advocate juicing as a detoxifying cleanse. Juice cleanses vary widely. Some are simply drinking sugary drinks all day long, but some are nutrient-dense powerful "meals" that can be very helpful. However, this takes knowledge-able planning to do it right. Juicing requires careful consideration to ensure proper intake of protein, healthy fats, fiber, and fruits and vegetables without taking in too much sugar. Consult your provider or an integrative nutritionist for help in planning a juice cleanse.

What we are talking about in this book is a collection of lifestyle habits that allow your body to detoxify naturally. When we have the right nutrients, sleep and fluids, **we are enhancing what our bodies do naturally.**

Be aware that there are few studies proving the efficacy of any particular detoxifying regimen. There is a plethora of literature, however, linking specific toxins with disease. So the problem is proven, even if there are many paths to a solution.

In general, it is a good idea to detox once or twice a year. This depends on your exposure, however. If you live directly under the flight path for the planes landing or taking off at an airport, or you work in a nail salon, you should detox more often.

Do not detox if you are pregnant or nursing. Also, if you have any chronic condition, as always, consult with your healthcare provider before taking any supplements.

Signs that you may benefit from a detoxification program:

- unexplained fatigue
- headaches
- brain fog
- bloating puffy eyes
- hormonal imbalance
- constipation
- rashes or skin irritation
- allergies
- numbness or tingling

If you are experiencing any of these symptoms, keep reading to learn the foundational strategies of detoxification.

*D*etoxification plans incorporate an "Elimination Diet". This is a diet that is free of certain common foods that are often difficult to digest. They cause intestinal inflammation, affect the immune system, and can cause systemic inflammation. By removing these foods from the diet, the body is not distracted by this inflammation. The body can then focus on detoxifying and removing stored toxins. Other foods should be eliminated because they are low in nutrients, high in sugar or bad fats, have preservatives or otherwise are just not nutritious. All of these need to be removed to improve gut health. Different detoxification programs may vary somewhat regarding which foods they allow, but they have more similarities than differences.

Foods to eliminate:

- Gluten or wheat
- Dairy (including yogurt)
- Corn
- Soy (tofu, tempeh, edamame)
- Commercial beef (grain-fed)

- Cured meats, sausages, cold cuts
- Pork
- Tuna
- Peanuts and peanut butter
- White potatoes
- Canned fruits and vegetables
- Alcohol
- Caffeine
- Sweets including honey, syrup, jam and agave (stevia is OK)
- Ketchup, barbecue sauce, or creamy salad dressings
- Snack foods like crackers, pretzels, and chips

This is when some might be thinking, "Oh, no! I can't eat anything good!" But that isn't true at all. There are a lot of healthy natural foods that **can** be eaten!

- Grass fed beef
- Free range chicken
- Wild caught salmon, cod, halibut or trout
- Venison
- Almond, coconut, rice or hemp milk
- Organic, cage-free eggs
- Quinoa, sweet potatoes*
- Rice, rice crackers*
- Gluten-free bread, gluten-free pasta, gluten-free steel cut oats*
- Organic beans, soaked and cooked or from BPA-free can
- Fresh or frozen fruits and vegetables. Eat a lot of them!
- Raw or dry roasted nuts and seeds
- Extra virgin olive oil, coconut oil, avocado and organic butter is usually OK
- Herbal tea or a cup or two of black tea if you need a little caffeine is fine

- Vegetable juice, coconut water

*If you want to lose weight, stay away from starchy carbs. But if not, you may eat small amounts if they are gluten-free.

The Dangerous Duo

Gluten and dairy are two foods that many of us just don't digest well. Why is that? First of all, gluten is a protein contained in wheat that is pretty much indigestible by humans. Gluten is often inflammatory and causes leaky gut, which can lead to gas, bloating, indigestion, reflux, abdominal pain, constipation or diarrhea.[69] Many of us already know we are sensitive to gluten, but many more haven't yet figured it out.

It is amazing to me as an integrative physician, how often people tell me they have "irritable bowel syndrome" with chronic bloating or diarrhea, and they have never tried to adjust their diet to see what is causing it. Irritable bowel syndrome is a ridiculous diagnosis. All it means is that something is causing inflammation. Somehow, mainstream medicine (doctors and patients alike) just accepts this as a real disease and then medicine is prescribed that only dulls the pain. It seems to me like a car that is knocking and sputtering, but the mechanic says, "Your car has Sputtering Disease. You'll just have to live with it. Put in earplugs and you won't hear it". Perhaps a better approach might be to figure out the root cause?

There are many who claim that gluten found in wheat products in Europe is not as inflammatory, and this may be true. Very commonly, wheat in the US is harvested with weed killer being sprayed on it in the fall, to uniformly dry the plants, so harvesting can be done efficiently.[70] I'm no agricultural expert, but there is definitely something different about wheat flour in the US compared to Europe.

Dairy is also problematic for many. The biggest issue is lactose intolerance. This is when your intestinal cells don't have enough lactase, the enzyme that breaks down lactose (milk sugar) into glucose and galactose. The lactose is fermented by your gut bacteria and gas develops. This causes bloating and diarrhea. About one-third of Americans have lactose intolerance.[71] However, for many people, the problem is even worse. Often we develop a sensitivity to casein and/or whey, the primary proteins in milk. Casein and whey can cause intestinal inflammation in a manner similar to gluten. This can contribute to systemic inflammation: brain fog, joint pain, fatigue, and even autoimmune diseases.

Food Sensitivities

Although gluten and dairy are probably the most common food sensitivities, there are plenty of other foods that one can be sensitive to. It varies widely and can be any number of other foods: fruits, vegetables, meat, nuts, etc.

There are food sensitivity blood tests that can be done, but in my experience, they are far from perfect. The results do not always correlate with symptoms, and occasionally a positive test for a food simply means that you eat it frequently and your immune system is fine with it, not that it is causing any problem.

Normally, when doing a detox, there is a shift in bowel function that can cause some bloating or change in stools. However, it usually improves after several days. If you have symptoms, ensure you are drinking a lot of water and eating high fiber foods. If you continue to have digestive issues after your detox, consult with your practitioner to discuss doing a food sensitivity test.

Organic or Not?

When it comes to produce, organic is often much better for us. Most produce in the US has detectable pesticide residues.[72] However, there is controversy as to what constitutes a safe and acceptable level. One study in children showed that within a few days of changing to organic produce, pesticides in the urine dropped dramatically. Then they returned within a few days of changing back to non-organic produce.[73]

However, organic produce is not always available, depending on where you live and what season it is. The best approach is to look up the "dirty dozen" on www.ewg.org. This is a list of the fruits and vegetables which have the highest risk of significant pesticide residue. For example, over 90% of strawberries have pesticides on them! Kale, apples and spinach are high on the list, too. For the dirty dozen, **always** spend a little more to get organic.

The "clean 15" is a nicer list. These are fruits and vegetables that do not need to be organic. For example, avocados and cabbage do not commonly have toxins in them. Check these lists every year; EWG does update them periodically.

EWG's 2020 Shopper's Guide to Pesticides in Produce ™

Higher Risk	Lower Risk
1. Strawberries	1. Avocados
2. Spinach	2. Sweet Corn
3. Kale	3. Pineapple
4. Nectarines	4. Onions
5. Apples	5. Papaya
6. Grapes	6. Sweet Peas (frozen)
7. Peaches	7. Eggplant
8. Cherries	8. Asparagus
9. Pears	9. Cauliflower
10. Tomatoes	10. Cantaloupe
11. Celery	11. Broccoli
12. Potatoes	12. Mushrooms
	13. Cabbage
	14. Honeydew
	15. Kiwi

Fun menus

This is a wonderful opportunity to have some fun! Set aside time every weekend to plan a menu for the week. This simple act will fill you with expectation instead of the dread you may feel at 5:15 driving home when you are hungry and realize you didn't plan anything.

I strongly encourage you to expand your repertoire. Add a variety of fruits to your grocery cart. Don't just get a bag of apples or bananas and call it a day...add something new! Buy a pineapple and cut it up. It takes a little time but it is so good! Purchase cherries if you don't normally buy them. Get some frozen organic berries and mix them with some coconut yogurt and stevia for a sweet but healthy dessert.

Eat plenty of green leafy vegetables (organic). Try baking kale chips or experimenting with new recipes for spinach. Learn how to roast Brussels sprouts or how to sauté broccoli and red peppers in extra virgin olive oil and pine nuts. Go online and search for vegetable recipes. You'll be amazed how good they can be when you mix several vegetables and try new seasoning. Get your spouse or your kids involved in meal planning. Do something new!

Just a word on starchy vegetables: corn and white potatoes should not be eaten during a detox. Corn is often an inflammatory food. White potatoes are too starchy and raise blood sugar quickly. Sweet potatoes are fine, as are carrots, but they do have a fairly high sugar content so watch your portion size.

Glycemic Load

When you are on a detox program, if you would like to lose a little weight, keep the glycemic load of your foods low. What is glycemic load? It is the ability of a food to raise blood sugar. High glycemic load foods include sugary drinks, baked goods, desserts, bread and pasta. Low glycemic load foods include non-starchy vegetables, berries, and fats. Foods in the middle include beans and high fiber grains like wild rice and quinoa.

This is important because food that spikes blood sugar harms the liver. Glucose triggers the release of insulin, the hormone that binds to glucose in the bloodstream and ushers it into the cell. It's like when your friend is inebriated, doing foolish things, and you gently put your arm around him and lead him inside and to bed. There he cannot get into trouble. When glucose is high and filling the bloodstream, it causes damage. It attaches itself to proteins and deforms them so they do not work (glycation). It can cause fatty deposits in the liver, which makes the liver sluggish and less able to do its job of detoxification. High glucose can cause inflammation in blood vessels, increasing the risk of a heart attack, a stroke, or dementia.

A healthy diet for everyone all the time is a relatively low glycemic diet. Fructose, found in high fructose corn syrup (HFCS), is particularly dangerous. It has the same damaging effects as glucose, but there is no insulin to bring it into cells. It is like the drunk who is making a mess but there is no friend to pull her inside. She runs around and messes everything up. HFCS does not trigger insulin release, so damage results. This is why you should never drink sugary drinks like sweet tea, juice or soda. They are empty calories and cause chronic disease. Just don't!

Antioxidant-rich foods

We all have heard that antioxidants are important but let's talk about why, and what foods are high in antioxidants.

"Oxidative stress" is a term in biochemistry that means that when oxygen combines with something else, a harmful substance can be formed. One name for these is "reactive oxygen species", or ROS. Another name is "free radicals". These ROS can damage cells and must be eliminated from each cell and then neutralized. Uncontrolled chronic oxidative stress can lead to inflammation and slowing of cellular metabolism which leads to organ dysfunction and symptoms of disease. Oxidative stress is linked to dementia, liver disease, diabetes, heart disease and cancer.

ROS are formed in higher numbers by things we do, such as smoking and drinking alcohol. (These are toxins, after all!) Pollutants also cause ROS to be formed. So we have control over some of this.

Many plant-based foods contain powerful compounds that neutralize ROS, so they are considered "antioxidants". Fruits high in antioxidants include most berries, but also grapes, oranges and cherries. Antioxidant vegetables include red cabbage, artichokes, spinach, kale, parsley, and beets. Also high in antioxidants are pecans, dark chocolate, coffee and green tea. These all have bioflavonoids and other phytonutrients that have high antioxidant capacity.

Detoxifying foods

Certain foods are particularly good for detoxification. They contain nutrients used in detoxing reactions in your cells. Sulfur containing vegetables help with sulfation, one of the liver Phase 2 reactions. Sulfur is also a critical component of glutathione, the "master antioxidant" of your body. Foods that provide sulfur include **onions, garlic, broccoli, eggs and nuts.**

Also, **cilantro** is known to help rid the body of heavy metals, phthalates and insecticides. Buy it fresh and organic, and add chopped cilantro to as many meals as you can!

Leafy greens like **kale and spinach** (organic) are just good for you, so make sure to include them. Cruciferous vegetables also enhance phase 1 liver detoxification. This includes **broccoli, cauliflower, and cabbage**.

Lastly, incorporate healing spices into your cooking. **Turmeric** or curry is well known to be anti-inflammatory. It actually is a supplement often included in detox kits! Add some to your eggs or your sautéed vegetables. Use **oregano** when you can; it helps the gut microbiome. **Ginger** is anti-inflammatory and makes a great hot tea. **Red pepper** can help with circulation. Get creative and spice it up!

. . .

A Word About Fiber

Many detox kits have fiber in the protein powders. It's there for a good reason: most Americans get very little fiber. We should get about 30-40 grams daily for optimal gut health, but most Americans get only around 15 grams daily. Fiber is so important! It feeds the healthy, good bacteria in the gut. It helps them grow which suppresses bad bacterial growth. Fiber also nourishes the enterocytes, which are the cells lining the intestine. It helps them stay healthy and absorb the right things while keeping the wrong stuff out. Some foods are also prebiotic, meaning they feed the good bacteria. Tomatoes, artichokes, bananas, asparagus and oats are prebiotic. Bananas are interesting. When green, they contain "resistant starch", which is not turned into glucose very well, but feeds the good bacteria. Once they are overripe, though, they have much more sugar.

Soluble and insoluble fiber are both important for good gut health. But you definitely need to drink plenty of water when you are increasing your fiber intake. If you don't, you can get bloated or constipated. Increase your fiber intake slowly if needed. And when you are done with your detox program, keep your fruit and vegetable intake high. This provides a lot of fiber and is good for you the rest of your life.

Cooking Tips

When you are cooking your food, do not use non-stick cookware with PFOA. Avoid using a microwave and never microwave food in plastic or on foam trays or plates. Also, make sure you do not overcook your food. When you char meat, cancer-causing compounds that are not good for you can be produced.[74] When you overcook vegetables, you decrease the fiber and lose other nutrient value. Lightly steamed veggies are very nutritious.

. . .

Hydration

Drink plenty of water! You should get about half your weight in ounces per day. So if you are 160 pounds, you should drink 80 ounces of water. Water is crucial for detoxification for several reasons. First, the body must be well hydrated for the kidneys to make urine, which is a major way toxins are eliminated. Water is also necessary for bowel motility, which is the other way toxins are removed. Water also is important on the cellular level. When you are dehydrated, your cells do not work as efficiently, so detoxification reactions may be slowed. Lastly, when you are dehydrated, you just don't feel well. You may have fatigue, brain fog, dizziness, headache and muscle cramps. So make sure you stay hydrated.

When you are drinking water, make sure it is filtered. Municipal drinking water may contain the very toxins we are trying to eliminate. Avoid bottled water, also. These plastic bottles have toxins in them that you don't need to drink. Pure, filtered water is what you need.

Consider drinking water with organic lemon juice in it. You can drink it hot or cold, but it can enhance digestion and mental clarity. Some people prefer to drink a tablespoon of apple cider vinegar in water once or twice a day. It doesn't taste quite as good, but the purported benefits of apple cider vinegar are pretty extensive. It certainly does seem to enhance digestion and may do much more.

Add a cup or two of hot green tea to your day. It's OK to add a little Stevia if needed. Green tea has bioflavonoids and antioxidants in it, and also has theanine. Theanine gives you a sense of calm focus, which often is helpful in the afternoon. The little bit of caffeine in green tea is generally harmless.

Plan your detox program for a time it will be easier to do. Consider events on your schedule, including holidays or travel. It also is much easier to detox when your family is supportive. It may not be easy to cook a gluten and dairy-filled meal for your children and then to eat a chicken breast and broccoli yourself. Try to get other family members to either eat what you are eating or to prepare and eat their meals separately from you to reduce temptation.

What if I get side effects?

Detox programs sometimes do cause flu-like symptoms the first few days, as your body adjusts to less sugar, less caffeine and your metabolism starts to adjust. Headaches, fatigue, mood swings and brain fog are fairly common. Drink plenty of water to reduce these symptoms. Get extra sleep and avoid stressful situations. Do not exercise strenuously; just taking a walk is fine. These symptoms usually only last 2-3 days and then you should start feeling a lot better.

How will I go without alcohol and caffeine?

If you are used to drinking alcohol every day, consult your healthcare practitioner for advice on how to safely remove alcohol from your diet. Abrupt cessation of more than a few alcoholic drinks per day can be dangerous.

Remember, that low alcohol intake (especially of organic wines) has some evidence of benefit.[75] However, less "clean" sources of alcohol (such as beer and cocktails) often have contaminants and sugar. Also, regular moderate to heavy alcohol intake is known to cause liver damage and cancer.[76] The liver turns alcohol into acetaldehyde, which is definitely toxic. So remember, even when not detoxing, it is best to not drink every day and to limit your intake. When you are detoxing, (just to state the obvious), don't drink a known toxin! It can make you feel ill and you can definitely live without it for a week or two.

In regards to coffee and tea, if you are used to drinking more than 2 cups of caffeinated beverages per day, it's better to simply limit yourself to one cup in the morning. This will help reduce caffeine-withdrawal headaches but should not interfere too much with your detox. If you can go without caffeine completely, that is even better. Any tea or coffee you drink should be organic.

Nutrition for Gut Health

Remember, that optimal intestinal function is crucial to detoxification. The liver and the kidneys both excrete toxins, and the intestine is a major way they are eliminated. The liver pushes toxins into the bile, which comes out through the bile duct into the upper portion of the small intestine.

This seems like it should be a clear path to the outside world, but the body has a pretty efficient mechanism for reabsorbing both good things and bad. This is called the enterohepatic circulation. A drug or toxin travels down the intestine, but can be reabsorbed along the way and then travels right back to the liver. It's like when you throw something in the trash but your spouse discovers it and brings it back in the house.

One way to reduce this effect during detoxification is to ensure proper bowel function. If you have slow bowel function, which usually causes constipation, the toxins that the liver and gallbladder dump into the intestine have much more time and opportunity to be reabsorbed. A normal transit time reduces this. Often the gut is called "Phase 3 detoxification". The liver completes phases 1 and 2, but the gut has to complete the final phase.

As previously mentioned, fiber is crucial for a healthy gut. So is drinking plenty of water. If you still struggle with constipation, magnesium citrate is often very helpful. The dose can be slowly increased until you are moving your bowels at least once a day. If you still struggle with constipation, talk to your healthcare provider.

Adding a binder can increase the efficacy of your detox. Commonly used binders include zeolite, bentonite clay, and activated charcoal. Binders do just that: they bind to toxins in the gut and prevent reabsorption, ensuring they are eliminated. They cannot be taken around food or other nutrients, however. Take them 30 minutes before eating or 2 hours afterward. Binders of various types have shown an affinity for organic pollutants, pesticides, herbicides, and mycotoxins (mold toxins).

Gut dysbiosis is when the mix of bacteria living in the intestine changes. This then affects gut cell function, nutrient absorption and overall health. When "bad" bacteria build up in the gut, inflammation develops which is commonly referred to as "leaky gut". Bacterial toxins called "endotoxins" can then be absorbed into the body across the inflamed, "leaky" gut cells. The most common type of endotoxin is lipopolysaccharides, or LPS. These are fragments of bacterial cell walls. When they escape the gut, they can cause widespread inflammation throughout the body.[77] Eating a healthy, whole food diet as we have been discussing goes a long way toward ensuring a healthy gut microbiome. You may also want to consider adding a probiotic to your fiber-rich, prebiotic supplying diet to improve your gut health. Naturally fermented foods like sauerkraut and kombucha contain probiotic bacteria that feed the gut so they are a natural probiotic.

In summary, your diet will have plenty of nutrient-dense, low sugar, high fiber plant foods with clean sources of protein and some healthy fat. You are eating to live, not living to eat. You will be fueling your body with powerful nutrients that give it the capacity to operate at peak efficiency. You will feel better!

After your Detox

Once your program is completed, be slow to reintroduce food types. This is especially true if you have had any symptoms of digestive issues. Gluten and dairy are difficult for many people, so I suggest only adding back one at a time for 3 - 4 days. This approach allows you to identify a food sensitivity. For example, if adding back cheese gives you bloating, this indicates lactose intolerance. If you add back gluten and get heartburn, you likely have gluten sensitivity. Your body will tell you what it can and cannot tolerate. If you are looking for those clues, and you listen to them, you can keep your gut in good shape.

If you simply return to eating gluten, dairy, sugar, and processed foods too quickly, you may notice your energy dropping or digestive issues. You will likely regain weight you had lost. Try to always come out of a detox with lifestyle habits that are a little bit better than before. This allows you to indulge once in awhile but overall maintain good health.

 Detoxification works because it addresses the needs of individual cells, the smallest units of human life

— PETER BENNETT ND

SUPPLEMENTS AND PRODUCT KITS

*M*ost pharmaceutical grade supplement companies have at least one "detox kit" which helps tremendously when detoxing. This typically is a box that contains a protein powder and other supplements and nutrients to enhance your success. There typically is also a booklet advising you on what to eat, what not to eat, and how to take the supplements.

These programs are all quite similar and any of them should work for you. If you have questions about how one compares to another, ask your healthcare practitioner.

The basics of a detox kit are:

- High quality protein powder to provide amino acids for detox support and protein for muscle maintenance
- Basic vitamins and minerals
- Specific detoxing supplements

When you do a detox kit, in general, you do not take any of your regular supplements. You usually do continue your prescription medications, however. Ask your provider for specific advice in your case.

Commonly used nutrients:

- Curcumin or turmeric
- N-acetyl cysteine or glutathione
- Milk thistle
- EGCG (from green tea)
- Alpha lipoic acid
- Calcium-D glucarate
- MSM
- Artichoke leaf extract
- Pomegranate fruit extract
- Sulforaphane
- Methionine, glycine and taurine
- Methyl B12 and methylfolate
- Resveratrol
- Zeolite or bentonite clay (binder)
- Activated charcoal (binder)

Most detox kits include the ingredients typically found in a multivitamin as well as added nutrients as above. Combinations vary, but overall, the effect is to assist the body in removing toxins while on a low-toxin diet.

Be careful to use products that are high quality and pharmaceutical grade, however. Some supplement companies do not use the highest quality ingredients, or they skimp on processes, so their product many not deliver these nutrients in levels that are effective. In general, look for a brand not sold openly in stores or on common reseller websites. The best brands with high quality products are generally sold only through qualified healthcare practitioners who can guide their patients in their proper use.

. . .

Chelation

If you have been diagnosed with heavy metal toxicity, talk with your practitioner about chelation therapy. While there are some over-the-counter binders that will remove heavy metals, and they often are very effective, sometimes stronger chelating agents are used. Commonly used chelators include EDTA, DMSA and DMSO. These should only be used with the guidance of a practitioner experienced in heavy metal chelation, as they can deplete mineral levels, and thus can be dangerous if not done properly.

SLEEP

*S*leep is so very important, and you may find that you need even more of it when you detox. Let's talk about what happens when you sleep, and you will understand how crucial it is that you get enough.

Sleep is still a pretty big mystery, but there is no question it is absolutely essential to life. Without sleep, the human body actually will die. Sleep deprivation has been used in history as a torture technique. So why do we believe that it is somehow OK to live with only 4 - 6 hours of sleep every night? Why do we stay busy at night and not get to bed until late, then drag ourselves out of bed in the morning, and drink coffee all morning to get going? Most of us underappreciate the power of good, full sleep and we all too easily make excuses for not getting enough.

What happens during sleep is extraordinarily complex, but we are starting to understand it more. We know the brain sorts through thoughts, memories and emotions, and then files important things into long term memory and forgets unimportant things. The memory sharpening effect of sleep has been studied in regards to learning. Just one night of sleep deprivation dramatically reduces the brain's ability to sustain attention during a task.[78, 79] (That's right, cramming for an exam was never a good idea. It still isn't).

The new interesting information about sleep is about how it cleans and restores the brain from a cellular metabolic standpoint. All cells, including brain cells, use nutrients and energy to do things. Certain things are made or processes are initiated, as the cell is designed to do, but there are waste products made in the cell. These include carbon dioxide and those reactive oxygen species, or ROS. These waste products must be cleared out.

Dr. Daniel Amen, a wonderful physician who is uniquely brilliant when it comes to brain health, talks about how the brain "takes a bath" at night when you sleep. Researchers have started to see evidence of an interesting phenomenon. When the brain goes into deep, non-REM sleep, the blood vessels in the brain shrink a little bit. This opens up some space between brain cells and the blood vessels. Fluid actually flows through this space as we sleep, flushing metabolic waste products out through the cerebrospinal fluid.[80] The brain literally does take a bath! This has an amazing regenerative effect.

Think about how terrible your brain felt if you have ever had a child who didn't sleep through the night for days or weeks on end. You likely were exhausted and, like my family used to say, "you can't think your way out of a paper bag." I suspect most of us parents know that feeling all too well!

But how do you feel on vacation, when you can sleep in and wake up with the sun and not an alarm? You feel great! The brain truly is much healthier with proper sleep. Research has shown that the vast majority of us need 7 - 9 hours of sleep a night.[81] Less than 7 solid, relatively uninterrupted hours can definitely decrease brain function.

So when we are talking about detoxing our bodies, that includes the brain. This is a great opportunity to focus on improving your sleep habits. As previously mentioned, when you detox, you often are much more tired and foggy than normal for a few days. Extra sleep is crucial at this stage. So do everything you can to get more sleep.

If you have sleep difficulties, now is a good time to really assess what else you can do. There are many reasons for sleep difficulties. The most common is stress or anxiety, but inflammation, blood sugar instability and hormonal imbalances do contribute. The other factor you cannot afford to ignore is your lifestyle habits. Sleep hygiene is very important. For example, you cannot watch suspenseful movies late at night or be active on social media (exposing your eyes to blue light) late at night and then expect your brain to go to sleep easily!

Good sleep hygiene is a foundation for optimal sleep:

- Keep a regular sleep schedule, whether it's a workday or not.
- Do not do stressful work in the evening.
- Dim the lights in the house 2 hours prior to bedtime.
- Turn off all screens 2 hours prior to bedtime. (TV, tablet, computer and phone). This is not easy, but sometimes is quite helpful.
- No screens in the bedroom. Charge your phone in another room so alerts do not disturb you.
- Keep your bedroom cool, dark and quiet. (turn down your thermostat – winter or summer – to no more than 68)
- Do not eat a large meal close to bedtime.
- No caffeine after 2 PM.
- Avoid alcohol. You may fall asleep a little quicker but

alcohol disrupts your sleep cycle to cause poor quality sleep that is non-restorative.
- Exercise regularly but not within 6 hours of bedtime.
- If you do not fall asleep within 20 minutes of going to bed, get up and do a quiet activity such as reading. Use your bed only for sleep and sex.

I can't sleep! What can I do?

Before we discuss supplements, first consider a few things:

- If you have daytime fatigue, please discuss with your practitioner whether you should have a sleep study done. Obstructive sleep apnea (OSA) is epidemic[82] and often silent. Many people with OSA have no idea they have it and they do not realize how absolutely crucial it is that it is identified and treated. If your sleep cycles are constantly being interrupted all night long by hypoxia (a drop in oxygen), you may wake up frequently and then will never feel energetic during the day. Home sleep studies are a very easy way to find out if this is an issue for you.
- When women transition through menopause, sleep disruption is common. Bioidentical hormones can often help your sleep quality, but they usually need to be used in conjunction with good sleep hygiene and supplements. Occasionally, prescription medications are still necessary.

Supplements

There are many supplements available to improve sleep. They typically have a number of ingredients in them that work together. Common ingredients include melatonin, GABA, theanine, valerian, magnesium, lemon balm, 5HTP, and passionflower.

However, when you are detoxing, I suggest you simply learn and plan your approach, but I do not recommend taking any new supplements for sleep. If you already are on one that works, then it is fine to continue to take it. But wait to try new supplements until after your detox. For now just make sure you are using good sleep hygiene and allowing plenty of time to sleep when you are tired.

When it comes to supplements, quality always matters! Any company can make a supplement for sleep, but the best supplements are made by companies that use high quality ingredients and produce a pharmaceutical grade product. Therefore, you often get what you pay for.

Everyone's brain is unique. Therefore, what works for you may not work for someone else. This simply requires that you try different products until you find a product that works for you. The process may take some time, but it will pay off!

Here is a list of my current favorite products for sleep. Ask your practitioner or see my website (www.integritywellnessmd.com) for a link to purchase them.

• Alpha-Theta Ultra PM™ from Biotics Research

• Alpha GABA PM® from Neuroscience

• Insomnitol™ from Designs for Health

• Liposomal Tranquinox Deep™ from NuMedica

• Melatonin SRT™ from Designs for Health

• CBD Synergies-SP from Quicksilver Scientific

In summary, do everything you can do with your daily routines and lifestyle habits to increase your chance of getting a good night's sleep. Work with your provider to address any medical issues that may be playing a part. Then start trying supplements. Once you find what works, this is important: it is much better to take it every night for awhile to re-train your brain to sleep well. Do not play the game of "should I take it or not?" Just take it every night to completely eliminate that stress. After a while, you can try to wean down your dose if you would like. But botanical ingredients are not at all bad for you, as long as the product is from a high quality company.

Also, remember: melatonin is a bioidentical hormone! If your body isn't making enough and you take some to supplement your brain levels, you are simply restoring a natural, optimal level of that hormone. There is absolutely nothing wrong with taking one of these natural products indefinitely.

Long term use of prescription medications such as Ambien®, Ativan® and the like have been associated with an increase in the risk for dementia in a few studies. This has not been definitively proven, but it is of some concern. We do know that these types of sleeping pills affect sleep cycles in an unnatural way, so sleep is not quite as restorative as natural sleep. So clearly, that is not a good long-term option. But the natural sleep supplements have no long-term risks. So at some point, consider giving them a try.

 True silence is the rest of the mind, and is to the spirit what sleep is to the body, nourishment and refreshment.

— WILLIAM PENN

STRESS

*S*tress. Who isn't stressed, right? It is obvious that most of us periodically have stress at work or at home. Physical conditions can add to your stress. So when your doctor says, "you need to detox", that may add to your stress even more!

Stress will affect your body's detoxification system, increasing the negative effect of toxins on your body. The more stressed you are, the more you may need to detox. And when you detox your body, I encourage you to detox your mind, your emotions and your schedule. Let's first talk about what stress does to your body.

Stress is Physical, Not Just Mental

Before we talk about reducing stress, we need to first understand the physical and medical effects of stress. Many people think it is just a psychological or mental feeling of frustration, depression, despair or anxiety. But stress is much more than just thoughts or feelings. It affects the entire body in ways you may not be aware of.

Stress generally results from situations where your expectations are not met. Perhaps things don't go like they should, or you fail to make progress toward a goal…that's frustrating. This creates emotional reactions that are accompanied by a change in neurotransmitters in the brain. There will be an increase in norepinephrine and epinephrine (adrenaline), the neurotransmitters that activate the "fight-or-flight" system, or sympathetic nervous system (SNS).

Fight or flight is when you suddenly experience a stressor. Your body is flooded with epinephrine, which prepares you to fight off the threat or run away. The SNS causes your pupils to dilate, your respiratory rate to increase, your heart rate to increase, and your muscles to tense up. Systems that typically work best when relaxed tend to get less blood flow, like the gut and hormones involved in reproduction.

Once the threat is gone, the SNS slows down and the parasympathetic nervous system (PSNS) takes over to relax you. The PSNS constricts pupils, slows breathing and heart rate, and relaxes your muscles. Your hormones and your gut work much better when the PSNS is in control.

We naturally go through our days with both the SNS and the PSNS working at different rates, so sometimes one will predominate. If you get up late, break a glass in the kitchen at breakfast, are slowed by a traffic jam and then spill your coffee in your car, then your SNS will be in overdrive before you even arrive at work!

Millions of us have lives that are full of stress. Our SNS is constantly being activated, like the gas pedal. The brake pedal, the relaxing PSNS, is weak and unable to balance the stressful SNS. When you detox your body, you need to consider your lifestyle and how balanced your SNS and PSNS are, for two reasons. First, if you don't address this during your detox, you will not be as successful at eliminating toxins and feeling better. Secondly, you will need to detox more often. The PSNS enhances detoxification and digestion, so if you cultivate stress-reducing habits in your lifestyle, you will naturally detoxify much better.

We also need to consider cortisol, the main stress hormone. Cortisol is made by your adrenal glands to help you deal with stress in the long haul. Adrenaline or epinephrine has effects right now, but cortisol has effects for hours to days. When you have chronic stress, your cortisol will be higher than it should. This can contribute to anxiety, mood swings, fluid retention, weight gain, diabetes and inflammation. If the stress continues, your cortisols can drop too low leading to exhaustion and depression. If you have chronic stress, talk to your integrative healthcare practitioner about options for testing and treating cortisol abnormalities that may persist after your detox.

Before your Detox:

Take a little time the day before you start your detox, or perhaps set aside time on day 1. Sit down with a cup of tea and really consider your lifestyle and how you currently handle stress. Make a list of the major stresses you have on one piece of paper, then make a list of how you are responding to stress. Write down what you are doing well and what you are doing wrong. Be honest with yourself! If you push yourself at work and leave later than you intend, then come home through rush hour traffic and are hungry and grumpy by the time you get home, admit it. Consider that perhaps leaving work a little earlier may circumvent a lot of those stressors. Conversely, if you are exercising regularly and it is helping you emotionally, you should feel good about yourself.

Please relax, though! Now is not the time to completely change all your bad habits. That would simply place more stress on you as you detox. But consider if there are a few things you can change during your detox. It doesn't have to be anything big, but pick something. For example, turn off the television at 8 PM and take a bath every evening. Buy some aromatherapy essential oils to have either for your home or in your bath. Schedule time to work on that project in the garage or to go fishing. Try to clear your calendar a bit to allow extra time for activities that are relaxing and enjoyable for you.

Journaling

Now is a good time to buy yourself a journal, if you don't already have one. Get a nice pen and enjoy a few minutes everyday alone with your thoughts. There is a verse in Proverbs that says, "without vision, the people perish" (Proverbs 29:18). Simply writing down what your goals are, where you are at and then developing a plan to achieve your goals, is very empowering.

Journaling actually has been studied in the medical community and has been shown to help with stress, mental health and with a number of medical conditions that cause chronic pain. **Journaling is an effective way to detoxify your mind.** When you write things down, it is similar to talking to a close friend or counselor. Simply unloading your thoughts and emotions to someone or on paper is truly therapeutic.

Often, emotional toxins have built up within our soul and we are not even aware of it. People who are always upset have inner conflict that has poisoned their thought life. These emotions are toxins that have festered because they have not been addressed.

One of the biggest emotional toxins is unforgiveness. Sometimes we do not forgive ourselves, so we demand even more from ourselves and others. In doing so, we alienate others and never live in peace with ourselves.

Sometimes we live with bitterness in our hearts toward someone else who has hurt us. It may be an abusive parent in the past, a former partner, or an adult son or daughter that has caused us great pain. This type of emotional toxin can negate all the physical things you can do. Take all the supplements you want and eat kale and cilantro, but if you are bitter in your heart, your body may not perform as it should due to inflammation or other metabolic issues and your emotional health will be an ongoing issue.

Go into your time of detoxing simply being honest with yourself about how you're doing emotionally. Decide on a few things you can improve upon.

During your detox:

While you are detoxing, especially the first few days, you may not feel your best so stress may be particularly difficult to deal with. Do your best to schedule your detox when stress will not make it more difficult. Plan on getting extra sleep, even if it means taking a 30-minute nap in the afternoon if your schedule allows. It's OK to nap!

Have strategies in place to mitigate stress. This can include quiet time for reading, watching a movie, working on a hobby, or other relaxing activities. This builds in pleasant activities you can look forward to which will reduce your adrenaline and cortisol, two stress hormones that can be detrimental.

Just a word here on self-nurture. This is a concept that most of us do not really think about. For those of us who work with customers, clients or anyone in the public in a service occupation, we take care of the needs of others all day long. We push our needs and wants aside to help others. This is not sustainable for the long haul. **We need time to take care of ourselves!**

Deep breathing exercises are very helpful. I recommend you set aside a few minutes every 3 - 4 hours to do this. In general, sit in a comfortable position and close your eyes. Draw in a slow deep breath through your nose, then exhale slowly and thoroughly through your pursed lips. Do this for a minute or two. Visualize nourishing, pure air coming in, and toxins being released.

If you have more time, consider meditation. Taking 10-20 minutes to practice the basics of quiet meditation is not only relaxing, but also can reduce inflammation and enhance cellular metabolic processes. If you are spiritual, pray as well. Many attest to the power of spiritual healing to cause mental and emotional healing, which definitely helps physical healing.

If there are certain activities you love to do but just never have time for, now is the time to do them! Schedule the time. What you never seem to find time for should be prioritized now. Maybe now is the time to plant those flowers in pots for your front porch. Or you really want to get the doghouse built for your puppy. Perhaps it's taking your son to play golf. Just **make** time every day to do something that brings you joy. This actually nourishes your mind and your soul, the same way nutrients work for your body. You deserve to be pampered and nourished.

Continue to journal during your detox. You may be surprised what you learn about your body. Perhaps you don't miss the wheat or the dairy, but not being able to have corn tortillas is very difficult (maybe your body craves corn but it's not good for you). You may realize that you really don't miss your nightly 1 - 2 beers or glasses of wine. Perhaps you have more energy because you are getting more sleep. As you journal both emotional thoughts and physical reactions, you may gain insight into how your body works. This is very valuable for the future.

In all of your time detoxing, please be gentle on yourself and be flexible with your routine. Realize that life will still go on, stressful situations may still arise, and you will have to adapt to them. Do not be afraid to say no to social invitations that would create busy stress. It's OK to slow down and be a little selfish. It's really not selfish, after all, **it's simply taking care of yourself.**

After Detoxing:

After your detox, I recommend you continue to employ self-nurturing techniques. Stress reduction is paramount in our world today, and your health depends on it. One of the biggest challenges is separating your stress from your reaction. Although they seem to be intertwined, they are not.

Consider Corrie ten Boom. She and her family lived in the Netherlands during Hitler's reign in World War II. They hid numerous Jews in their home, saving their lives, but taking great risk for their own. She and her sister ended up in a concentration camp and her sister perished there. Somehow, Corrie survived and lived to tell her story. She was a woman of great faith. She once said, "happiness isn't something that depends on our surroundings. It's something we make inside ourselves." Think about that for a moment...it's very powerful.

The Serenity Prayer is worth remembering each and every day. Here is a portion:

> *"God give me grace to accept with serenity*
> *the things that cannot be changed,*
> *courage to change the things*
> *which should be changed,*
> *and the wisdom to distinguish*

the one from the other.
Living one day at a time,
enjoying one moment at a time;
accepting hardships as the pathway to peace."

— REINHOLD NEIBUR

If you are a person of faith, I encourage you to look up the whole text. It is quite inspiring. But for all of us, it is truly a challenge to view our difficulties as something positive.

Things happen. Bad, painful, tragic things happen. This book is being written in 2020, the year of a pandemic that has caused much suffering. But this is not the first time in history our civilization has suffered greatly, and it will not be the last.

Remember, no matter how stressful your situation is, someone is dealing with something far worse. Know that "this too shall pass". The vast majority of our stresses get better over time, so we need to be on guard for persistent toxic emotions.

Bear in mind, that stress is not all bad, though. Without some stress, we would lead very boring lives. Hans Selye, the early researcher on stress, wrote, "Stress is the spice of life. Without stress, life lacks excitement, challenge and a sense of adventure." So stress itself isn't bad.

What hurts us about stress psychologically and physically is **our response** to the stress. The literature in psychology has demonstrated that our reaction to a stressful event dramatically sets our body on course for how much of an effect the stress will have.

Let's just say your car breaks down on the way to work. You can react positively, by being thankful you weren't in a car accident, and that it is a fixable problem. Yes, it is inconvenient, but fixable within a few days. You can call your boss and even if he or she is upset, you can choose to not allow it to sour your attitude. You can practice gratefulness all day. This attitude will help you focus on the steps necessary to solve the problem.

On the other hand, you can get upset and allow it to ruin your day. You can feel sorry for yourself, get angry that you have to deal with another problem, get frustrated that you are inconvenienced, and sulk. If you choose to do this, you will not only have a sour personality all day, but you can actually make yourself sick. Your adrenaline and cortisol can go up causing you to get a headache, an upset stomach (stress causes leaky gut), or even come down with an infection of some sort.

Never forget a very important principle:

Although you have little control over what happens to you, you have complete control over your response!

You choose what you say. You choose whether to indulge in self-pity. You choose how you will affect others by your mood. You choose how you will solve your problem. It's all up to you! Keep your mind clear of emotional toxins. Life is much better that way.

DETOX YOUR SCHEDULE

*T*here are other aspects to detoxification that go beyond food, cellular toxins and even stress. As an integrative physician, my job is to look at health in a holistic fashion. You also need to realize that if you do a perfect detox, you are at risk for going backward if you don't ensure your whole life is detoxed is all ways.

One common thing that is toxic to our health is our schedule. Time management is a lofty but necessary goal. We all have to juggle a lot of demands on our time. We use electronic calendars to keep us on track. Alarms and reminders keep us focused on the next task. Parenting and work demands are constant the whole day long. Many of us overcommit and then what is the result? STRESS. We have already talked about stress, but let's talk about time management a bit.

Think for a moment about a broad but important question:

What is your purpose in life?

This is a deep question and everyone has different answers. Then consider the following two questions:

1. **What keeps you from your purpose?**
2. **What steals your joy?**

Life coaches usually start with these concepts. They help you build your life and your habits around the central pillar of what your purpose is. Fulfilling your purpose should give you joy!

I love the book "Manage Your Time To Reduce Your Stress" by Rita Emmett. She encourages us to seek out the things that we value, reach for realistic goals, and eliminate activities that are unnecessary, all while incorporating self-nurture.

Consider what I call Time Toxins:

- Unimportant but urgent issues
- Obligations
- Not enforcing boundaries
- Social media and television
- Email
- Procrastination
- Perfectionism
- Boredom
- Isolation

Urgent Issues:

For many of us, it's the first that chews up much of our time. When small things come up at work, such as a coworker asking us a question, it may only take a minute or two. But it interrupts our thoughts and our productivity. When that happens 20 times in a day, overall efficiency goes down and frustration sets in. If all those questions could happen all together in a 30 minute meeting, we would be more productive and feel less stressed.

Obviously, many jobs exist to address customer issues. Retail, call centers, and many more are there to do just this. But if you have a job that requires focus and sustained attention, try to limit interruptions.

Multitasking is common, but really isn't good for productivity. When you are focused on one thing, you will do a better job. When you are conferencing with your attorney or your financial adviser, do you want them answering texts or emails or calls while they talk with you? Would you want your surgeon dictating a text reply or a message to office staff about someone else when he or she was operating on you? No and no! Stay focused and your stress will go down. Your moods will improve.

The best example of distractions in an office job is the ping of new emails coming in. Turn this off! How many times have you gone down the rabbit hole of "I'll just deal with a few emails now then get back to my work", then 30 minutes later you are still working on emails? Schedule time to handle emails and then leave them alone the other times. This is not easy, I know, but it will make you more efficient.

The corollary to this is working at home in the evening. Many people just feel the need to finish up work on the computer at night and will respond to emails after supper. If your job does not absolutely require this, don't do it! You will be much more productive if you just start a little earlier the next day. Your evening will be relaxing, and will therefore make you healthier.

Obligations:

Detoxify your schedule. If you are running your children to different activities every day of the week while working a full time job, you're just too busy. It's OK to say no to some things! Sometimes family members pressure you to do things that you really don't have time for. Do not say yes to a time obligation unless you can do it with a good attitude and it will not create stress for you. Give your time with joy and a generous spirit, not out of a sense of obligation. There will be a difference in how your body responds. One produces health and joy, but the other produces resentment and inflammation.

Media:

For years I called Facebook a "time-sucker". I saw people spend hours on Facebook every day so I didn't have an account for years. I simply refused to waste my time! When I did get an account, I did it because it helped me connect with relatives that lived across the country. I used it to connect relationally but learned quickly that there are many "quicksand" traps that will suck you into strife in a flash. Social media has become a mine-field. One wrong comment and boom! You can be vilified and destroy a relationship. Social media can be as toxic as a poison. I have seen patients so upset about what they read on social media that it comes into the exam room. They are depressed, angry, not sleeping and have more digestive issues. If you use social media at all, limit your time on it and use it for the good it can bring: connecting and encouraging others. Don't drink the poison.

Television is another "time-sucker". Many of us are guilty of binge-watching a show on TV. Sometimes our televisions are on all day Sunday with football games. Do you realize, though, that some people have the TV on every moment they are home and awake?

We were on vacation once in a rented cabin in the mountains with several other couples. We had a fantastic time! That vacation was so rejuvenating, and one reason was because I saw no television for 4 days. When our family visits my mother, we tease her because she has the cheapest cable subscription in her town. She has no ESPN, no cable news, and no kids' channels (our kids lamented that when they were young). But you know what? Other than football games, we don't watch TV when we visit. It is great! We play card games, talk, and really connect. Try it at home. Try a whole day of no TV. It truly is revitalizing.

Perfectionism:

If you're anything like me, you like to do things right—*exactly* right. Imperfect just isn't acceptable...but this will only cause you stress! When you feel like you have to be perfect, you will spend a lot more time on something, and you probably will waste time. This is self-imposed stress which is toxic. I bought a water bottle last year that says "Perfectly Imperfect". Every time I look at it, I remember that being imperfect is just fine. It actually is much healthier than being perfect!

Helen Keller (who knew a thing or two about imperfection) said,

 Being happy doesn't mean everything's perfect. It means you've decided to see beyond the imperfections!

Isolation:

If you are alone, you need to make special effort to connect to other people. Sometimes, being alone or retired is particularly challenging when it comes to time management. Have you ever had what I call a "crash day?" I've had days where I just didn't have the energy to do anything. I realize that I need to relax and do nothing, so that's what I do. But then the next day, I feel better and get back to a normal pace.

If you live alone or are retired, you may find that not having a schedule makes it harder to get things done. You may dawdle in getting started on a task, simply because you can. If you live alone, there is no one there to keep you accountable. Lack of motivation leads to fatigue, lethargy, and then isolation. Isolation can lead to depression. Manage your time wisely, even when you have fewer demands on it. Stay purposeful with your time and invest it wisely.

Stay connected to others as much as you can! Make the effort to reach out to others and live life with them. Keep doing things that give you joy. Volunteer and give to others who need a helping hand. There is much joy in giving, especially giving our time to others. Avoid the toxins of boredom, sluggishness and apathy.

In summary, make sure you know your values, your goals, and what brings you joy. Make sure your activities move you in that direction.

 When you spend more time doing what is not important to you, and little or no time on what is truly important to you, the result is usually stress, frustration and a sense of inadequacy.

— RITA EMMETT

Ditch these time toxins. Spend your time **intentionally** on things that give you peace, fulfillment and joy!

DETOX YOUR STUFF

*H*ave you seen any of the television shows about hoarders? Wow! I have seen a few episodes, but after awhile, I just couldn't watch any more. People who are compulsive hoarders have a psychological issue where they attach a high emotional value to an object, and then they cannot let it go without suffering emotional pain. It's hard for me to understand.

Many couples are like my husband and I. He's the keeper, and I'm the tosser. This has gotten me in trouble more than once! I grew up without a lot of tangible items that meant much to me, and I've had to move more than a few times, so I am comfortable with donating something and replacing it. My husband, however, feels strongly attached to certain items. An object will remind him fondly of an old friend, good memories from college, or a place he used to live. It is much harder for him to part with certain objects.

Neither of these approaches is good or bad; it's just how we are wired. But there is a point where objects create psychological stress. In our attempts to control our environment (collecting items), we actually lose control over our environment (the objects control us).

Without getting into the psychology too deeply, which is complex, I would suggest that you simply ask yourself whether you have any objects that are causing emotional stress. If you have a desk piled high with stuff making it unusable, and then you work at the kitchen table, which gets cluttered, and then you have to eat dinner on the couch...well, you might be increasing your stress.

Objects in our homes and office should be both functional and in keeping with an atmosphere of peace. If your office is arranged in a way that makes you inefficient, you will get frustrated. Rearrange things. Similarly, if your clutter reminds you every day of your failures, clean it up! This is an emotional toxin that is preventable and fixable.

If you struggle with clutter, start small. Only tackle one room at a time, and do not try to do it all in one marathon session on a Saturday. Set a timer for 1-2 hours and work diligently sorting through objects. It is easiest to clear all the clutter from a desk or area of the room, by moving it all aside. Yes, move EVERY-THING! Now, clean the floor or surfaces, and then you are ready to start sorting. Make three piles: Keep, Donate or Toss. You'll probably be amazed how much ends up in the donate or toss piles.

Once you have everything sorted, take a break. This is not easy, and you need to unfocus for a few minutes to relax. If you still have time and energy to keep going, the next task is organizing the items you are keeping in a functional way. This applies to clothing, kitchen items or home office contents. If you need to do the organizing and putting away another time, that is fine! You do not want to rush through this step if you are tired or struggling emotionally.

Once you are done with that area, congratulate yourself! You can clean out an entire home with this process but it takes time. Allow yourself the time you need, but don't let yourself procrastinate. Set times for this task and stick to them. Detox your house. You can do it!

EMOTIONAL TOXINS

*B*efore we move on, we need to consider emotional toxins. Day-to-day stress is certainly toxic to our mood, our energy and our mental health. However, there are deeper, more dangerous toxins that, if not handled properly, will ultimately make us sick.

People

Some people are simply annoyingly selfish, but some are emotionally broken, which comes out as anger. Toxic relationships are complicated, because there usually are compelling reasons to stay connected. Often it's a family member, a spouse, a child, or even a co-worker or boss. Sometimes it's easy to separate from someone who is toxic, but if you're related to them, it's much harder.

Have you ever had a lopsided friendship? You know, the type of friend who only talks about him or herself? I have, and it gets old very quickly. Invest your time and your friendship with people who appreciate you and care about you. This will bring emotional healing when times get rough, rather than create resentment, which is a very powerful emotional toxin.

Abusive relationships vary from obvious to subtle. No matter how minor the abuse is, it is more toxic than many of the chemicals we discussed earlier. Hidden emotional pain can cause a great deal of disease and suffering. And even worse, because it is hidden, there is no one by your side to console you or cheer you up. Pain plus isolation is deadly. If you are struggling with any toxic relationships, I urge you to seek help. Seek counseling, and if you belong to a church or synagogue, seek spiritual counsel. You'll be so glad you did.

Anxiety

It seems nowadays that everyone has some degree of anxiety. We live in a day and time where life is completely unpredictable. Economic ups and downs, crime, job loss, political upheaval, and disease are constant worries. There are three strategies for dealing with anxiety:

1. Psychological
2. Spiritual
3. Integrative medical

If you truly struggle with anxiety, there are great books you can read to give you strategies on dealing with anxiety. Meditation, yoga, and prayer all have shown benefit in reducing anxiety. Counseling also is helpful. Keep in mind that anxiety is two main things: being uncomfortable, and being fearful.

Uncomfortable is what you feel at a cocktail party when your date goes off to talk business to a coworker, and you don't know anyone there. Uncomfortable is when you have to give a presentation to your boss. Uncomfortable is when you're sitting at the table at the restaurant alone, waiting for the other person to arrive, and others are looking at you.

When most of us feel uncomfortable, we immediately want to make that feeling go away. We pick up our phone and scroll through something, or maybe we just escape to something that feels safer. We calm ourselves by not dealing with being uncomfortable. A better approach is to feel the discomfort, and learn to tolerate it.

The deeper level of anxiety is fear. We fear making mistakes in the presentation and having our coworkers or boss think less of us. We fear what others will think of us. We fear failure.

One of the best TED talks I have heard was by Tim Ferriss. He gives a powerful argument for doing what he calls "fear setting". Look it up online and watch it. In essence, he says you should write down exactly what you are afraid of. Once you list all your fears, ask yourself "What are the benefits of partial success?" Then ask yourself, "What is the cost of inaction?" Just the first part is very empowering. When you honestly admit what you're afraid of, you realize WHY you're feeling anxious. But the second part is quite educational, also. So often, we don't move forward out of fear of failure. But often, we achieve at least partial success, which puts us way ahead. The final thing we usually don't allow ourselves to consider, is that there is a significant price to pay for inaction.

From an integrative medicine standpoint, anxiety is often related to gut inflammation. We talk about the "gut-brain connection" frequently. Did you know that most of your serotonin, the feel-good brain neurotransmitter, is made in the gut? Eating a whole food, anti-inflammatory diet helps your brain work better.

Anxiety and depression are emotional toxins that color our lives in a pervasive way. Do what you can to limit their effect on you.

Chasing Success

Many people are type A, "work-a-holics", who simply can't slow down until they achieve their next goal. Once they reach that goal, there's the next. And the next. It used to be mostly the men who worked long hours at the expense of family time. Now it's not limited by gender at all. Women work just as hard to achieve success in their careers while also juggling family duties. This creates enormous stress.

Interestingly, in the past decade, we've seen a trend away from large homes and lavish lifestyles, to more people downsizing. My husband loves to watch shows on TV about "tiny homes". I admire these people greatly, but I just don't know if I could quite do that. But do you really need a 5000 square foot home after all the kids are grown? Do you need to live in that exclusive area of town where all the homes are grand and expensive? Are you trying to appear successful to impress others?

Don't misunderstand; there is absolutely nothing wrong with having a big house or wealth. If you are wealthy and use it properly, it can be a tremendous blessing to your family and to others. But some of the wealthiest (and happiest) people I've known are the ones in overalls or T-shirts and jeans...they aren't the ones trying to impress anyone. The problem comes when you feel compelled to impress others. You are constantly reaching for more and more, yet never satisfied. Attention and accolades from others is addictive. This is an emotional toxin. Literature is full of examples of rich men who were miserable creatures...their addiction to success ruined them.

Live life fully and learn to be content. I like to live *contented* in every situation, even though I may not be *satisfied*. There is a difference. You can be perfectly content in a situation that you do not have satisfaction in yet.

> *Not that I speak in regard to need, for I have learned in*
> *whatever state I am, to be content.*

— PHILIPPIANS 4:11

Resist being emotionally addicted to success. When you stop chasing wealth, attention or acclaim, it seems to find *you*. And you will have much less anxiety.

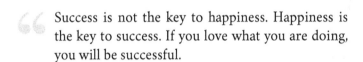 Success is not the key to happiness. Happiness is the key to success. If you love what you are doing, you will be successful.

— HERMAN CAIN

ENHANCING YOUR DETOX

So far, we have discussed food, hydration, nutrients, sleep and stress. However, there are other modalities you can add to your routine to enhance your health.

Baths and Sauna

Although we haven't talked much about detoxification through sweat, some toxins are definitely secreted into the sweat glands. Therefore, when you sweat, this can help reduce toxin load. You can do this by simply taking a hot bath on a regular basis. Add some Epsom salts to the water and perhaps some essential oils, and enjoy the aromatherapy.

Another popular method of detoxification is infrared (IR) sauna. These saunas can be purchased for home use but often are found in holistic practitioner's offices. IR saunas work by heating your body, not the air around you. IR can improve circulation, reduce inflammation and assist with detoxification through sweating. Consult your holistic practitioner to learn more.

. . .

Exercise

Exercise is important all the time, but you do need to be careful when detoxing. The first few days most people do well with just walking and nothing strenuous. After that, you can do moderate exercise but should not do particularly heavy workouts. You want to improve your circulation and energy levels, but you do not want to do tissue damage that causes inflammation.

Clean air

During your detox and from now forward, pay attention to the air you breathe. Most people are unaware how many pollutants are in the air, especially in the city or near industrial plants. Perhaps in rural Wyoming the air is safer, but no matter where you are, you should know whether there are any factories or industries nearby that are affecting air purity.

Since it is difficult to avoid airborne pollutants, air filters are strongly recommended in your home and your workplace. A number of companies make HEPA filters that not only **filter** but also **purify** the air. The filter eliminates large particles like animal dander and pollen, but the purifying mechanism destroys VOC's (volatile organic compounds) and other small sized pollutants that pass right through a simple filter.

It is obvious to most of us, but do not smoke and do not spend time in a building where smoking occurs. Secondhand smoke and even the leftover smell from a smoker are irritating to your system and contain toxins.

RECIPES

*H*ere are some healthy recipes using clean, anti-inflammatory ingredients. All of them are gluten and dairy-free. Make sure you purchase organic ingredients when you can. Enjoy them all…including the desserts!

APPETIZERS AND SALADS

Baja Salmon Avocado Dip

2 avocados, halved

14-16 oz wild caught salmon, cooked and flaked

1 tbsp lemon juice

1 tbsp lime juice

1 tbsp taco seasoning or chili powder

1 cup tomatoes, chopped

1 cup onion, chopped

2-3 jalapeños, chopped

½ cup fresh cilantro, chopped

Cut avocados in half and scoop out avocado, leaving ¼" rim for shell. Set shells aside. Dice avocado and mix with all other ingredients. Fill avocado shells with mixture. Serve with hot sauce and gluten-free crackers, celery sticks, or carrots. (Note: when not detoxing, this is excellent with tortilla chips but corn should be avoided during a detox).

Greek Salad

2 English cucumbers, cut into ½" cubes

2 lb tomatoes, cut into ½" cubes

1 medium red onion, chopped, then rinsed and drained

1 1/3 cups coarsely chopped parsley

1 1/3 cups drained pitted kalamata olives, halved if large

½ cup extra virgin olive oil

½ cup lemon juice

1 ½ tsp oregano

Salt and pepper

Mix cucumber, tomatoes, onion, parsley and olives. In another bowl, mix the olive oil, lemon juice and oregano. Add dressing to vegetables and add salt and pepper to taste.

Mexican Black Bean Salad

1 cup chopped cilantro

½ cup chopped red onion

3 Roma tomatoes, chopped

2 jalapeños, chopped

1 red pepper, chopped

2 tsp minced garlic

2 cans organic black beans, rinsed and drained

2 large avocados, chopped

Dressing:

1 tbsp salt

1 tbsp cumin

6 tbsp fresh lime juice (from 3 limes)

5 tbsp olive oil

2 tbsp apple cider vinegar

Mix cilantro through black beans. Mix dressing. Just prior to serving, add dressing and avocado.

(Note: 1 lb corn in a few tbsp oil, roasted at 450° for 20 min, makes this salad even prettier. However, corn should be avoided during a detox).

Fajita Salad

2 medium boneless, skinless chicken breasts, cut in half horizontally

2 cups sliced bell peppers (mixture of colors)

1 head Romaine lettuce, chopped

1 avocado, sliced

4 tbsp olive oil

4 tbsp lime juice

½ cup cilantro, chopped

2 cloves garlic, minced

1 tsp brown sugar

1 tsp ground cumin

1 tsp salt

Whisk the marinade ingredients (olive oil through salt) together in a medium bowl. Pour half of the mixture onto the chicken breasts and coat them well. Cover and refrigerate for at least 30 min (up to 24 hrs is OK). Reserve the rest of the marinade.

Heat a large heavy duty skillet or pan to medium-high heat for 2 minutes. Add a teaspoon of oil to the pan and then add chicken breasts. Cook 4-5 minutes per side or until cooked through. Remove from pan and cool for 5 min on cutting board, then chop or slice. Add the bell pepper slices to the pan and cook on high for 1-2 min.

Divide the lettuce into two salad bowls. Top each salad with half the chicken, bell peppers and sliced avocado. Serve with the remaining marinade as dressing.

BREADS

Gluten-free Apple Cinnamon Muffins

1 ½ cup applesauce

1/3 cup melted butter

2 eggs

½ cup sugar

1 tsp vanilla

½ tsp salt

1 ½ cup gluten-free flour (King Arthur Measure-for-Measure is best)

1 tsp baking soda

½ tsp baking powder

1 tbsp cinnamon

Topping:

¼ cup brown sugar

2 tbsp sugar

½ tsp cinnamon

1/3 cup gluten-free flour

2 tbsp melted butter

Mix applesauce, butter and eggs. Add sugar, vanilla and salt, then add flour, baking soda, baking powder and cinnamon. Mix well. Mix dry ingredients for topping, then add butter and mix. Fill muffin tins with batter and top with crumb topping. Bake at 350° for 20 minutes. Makes 12.

Gluten-Free Keto Bread

½ cup melted butter

3 tbsp coconut oil, liquid or melted

6 large eggs

1 1/3 cup almond flour

2/3 cup coconut flour

1 tsp baking powder

½ tsp xanthan gum

½ tsp salt

Break eggs into mixer bowl and whisk. Add remaining ingredients and mix until dough is formed. Spread in greased 9x5" loaf pan. Bake at 350° for about 40 minutes, until top is browned.

Gluten-Free Banana Bread

1 cup sugar

1 stick butter, softened

2 eggs

3 bananas, mashed

1 tbsp almond milk

½ tsp cinnamon

2 cups gluten-free flour (King Arthur Measure-for-Measure works best)

1 tsp baking soda

1 tsp baking powder

1 tsp salt

Mix the sugar and butter until smooth. Add eggs and mix. Add bananas, almond milk and cinnamon. Mix dry ingredients together in a bowl, and then slowly add to banana mixture. Bake in loaf pan at 350° for 60-70 minutes.

SOUPS

Slow Cooker Chicken Enchilada Soup

1 onion, diced

3 cloves garlic, mashed

1 red pepper, diced

1 jalapeño, minced

8 oz tomato sauce

1 tbsp chili powder

1 tbsp chipotle pepper in adobo sauce, chopped

2 tsp cumin

1 tsp garlic powder

1 tsp onion powder

1 tsp white wine vinegar

1 tsp sea salt

½ tsp oregano

3 cups chicken broth

1 lb free-range chicken breasts

Sauté onion, garlic and pepper in skillet in olive oil. Mix tomato sauce through chicken broth. Place into slow cooker with chicken breasts. Cook on low 6-7 hours or until chicken is done.

Pumpkin Chili

2 lb grass-fed ground beef

1 medium onion, chopped

1 cup canned pumpkin

1 (20 oz) can diced tomatoes

1 (16 oz) can kidney beans, drained

1 (12 oz) bottle chili sauce

1-2 tbsp chili powder

2 tsp pumpkin pie spice

1 tsp brown sugar

1 ½ tsp salt

1 tsp black pepper

1-2 cups water

Brown ground beef and onion. Drain any excess grease. Add remaining ingredients and mix. Add enough water to desired consistency. Bring to a boil and simmer for 1 hour.

MAIN DISHES

Keto Korean Beef Bowl

Cauliflower rice:

1 tbsp olive oil

1 lb cauliflower (frozen riced or freshly riced)

½ tsp sea salt

1/8 tsp black pepper

Beef:

1 tbsp olive oil

1 lb grass-fed ground beef

½ tsp sea salt

4 cloves garlic, minced

¼ cup light soy sauce

¼ cup beef broth

2 tsp sesame oil

½ tsp ground ginger

¼ tsp crushed red pepper flakes

Heat the olive oil in a large wok over medium-high heat. Add riced cauliflower. Season with salt and pepper. Sauté for 3-5 minutes until cooked through. Cover to keep warm and set aside.

In a small bowl, whisk the soy sauce, broth, sesame oil, ginger and red pepper flakes. Set the sauce aside.

Turn heat to medium-high. Add another tablespoon olive oil to the wok. Add the ground beef and sea salt. Cook for about 8-10 minutes until browned. Make a well in the beef and add the minced garlic. Sauté for about a minute, until fragrant, then mix into the beef.

Pour the sauce over the beef. Bring to a simmer, then reduce heat and simmer for 3-4 minutes, until the sauce is thickened.

Divide the cauliflower rice among plates. Top with ground beef. Garnish with chopped green onion, sesame seeds and/or sliced cucumber.

Beef Slaw

1 lb grass-fed ground beef

1 tbsp + 1 tsp extra virgin olive oil

1 tsp garlic, minced

Salt and pepper to taste

3 ½ cups shredded cabbage

½ cup chopped green onion

Sauce:

½ tsp sugar

½ tsp ginger paste or freshly grated ginger

1 tsp white vinegar

2 tbsp soy sauce (gluten-free)

1 tsp chili paste or hot sauce

In a large skillet, brown the ground beef and garlic in 1 tbsp olive oil. Season with salt and pepper. Drain any excess grease. In a bowl, mix sauce ingredients. In the skillet, heat 1 tsp olive oil. Add cabbage and green onion. Stir fry until cabbage is slightly wilted and tender. Stir in the sauce and add the meat. Serve hot.

Slow Cooker Chili Verde

2 – 7 oz cans diced green chilis

1 – 20 oz package of ground free range turkey (or grass-fed beef)

2 cups chopped onions

1 tsp crushed or minced garlic

2 cups chopped zucchini

2 cups chopped tomatillos

½ tsp cumin

¼ tsp black pepper

1 tsp sea salt

½ tsp dried oregano

1/8 tsp cayenne pepper

2 cups chicken broth

1 tbsp grapeseed oil

Sauté garlic and zucchini in grapeseed oil. Add turkey and brown. Transfer to crock pot with remaining ingredients. Cook on low for 4 hours.

Keto Chicken and Vegetables

4 chicken breasts (free-range)

2 tbsp olive oil

1 lemon, juiced and zest rind

1 tsp garlic powder

1 tsp salt

Black pepper

1 red onion cut into wedges

1 lemon cut into wedges

8 oz fresh green beans

1 red pepper sliced

Put the chicken in a bowl. Add 1 tbsp oil, lemon zest, half the lemon juice, garlic, salt and pepper. Mix and marinate for 30 min. Preheat oven to 400°. Place the chicken, onion and half the lemon wedges on a sheet pan. Bake for 20 minutes. While baking, place green beans, red pepper, remaining oil and remaining lemon juice in a bowl and mix. Add this vegetable mixture around the partly cooked chicken. Back for another 15 minutes and serve with remaining lemon wedges.

Cauliflower Fried Rice with Chicken

1 tsp grapeseed oil

2 large eggs

3 pieces green onion, thinly sliced

1 tbsp ginger, grated

1 tbsp garlic, minced

1 lb boneless, skinless chicken (free-range)

½ cup red pepper, diced

1 cup snow peas, trimmed and halved

4 cups cauliflower rice

3 tbsp soy sauce (gluten free brand)

Heat 1 tsp oil in wok or large skillet over high heat. Add eggs to pan, stir and cook. Remove cooked eggs from pan and set aside. Add 1 tbsp oil to the pan with green onions, ginger and garlic; cook, stirring, until onions have softened, about 30 seconds. Add chicken and cook, stirring, for 1 minute. Add pepper and peas; cook, stirring, until just tender, 2-4 minutes. Add the remaining 1 tbsp oil to the pan; add cauliflower rice and stir until beginning to soften, about 2 minutes. Return the chicken mixture and eggs to the pan; add soy sauce and stir until well combined. Garnish with green onions.

Chicken and Veggie Frittata

1 cup broccoli florets

½ cup fresh mushrooms, sliced

2 green onions, finely chopped

8 oz free-range chicken, cubed

4 large eggs

2 egg whites

¼ cup water

¼ cup Dijon mustard

½ tsp Italian seasoning

¼ tsp garlic salt

½ cup chopped tomatoes

In a skillet, sauté the broccoli, mushrooms and onions in olive oil until tender. Add chicken and heat through. Remove from heat and keep warm. In a mixing bowl, beat eggs, water, mustard, Italian seasoning and garlic salt until foamy. Add tomatoes and broccoli mixture. Pour into a greased shallow 1½ quart baking dish. Bake at 375° for 22-27 minutes, or until a knife inserted in the center comes out clean.

Italian Skillet Chicken and Mushrooms

4 large free range chicken breasts, cut into ¼" thin cutlets

1 tbsp dried oregano

1 tsp salt

1 tsp black pepper

½ cup gluten-free flour (King Arthur Measure-for-Measure works best)

8 oz baby bella mushrooms, sliced

14 oz grape tomatoes, halved

2 tbsp chopped garlic

½ cup white wine

Juice freshly squeezed from ½ a lemon

¾ cup chicken broth

Handful of baby spinach

Pat chicken cutlets dry. Season on both sides with ½ tbsp. oregano, ½ tsp salt and ½ tsp pepper. Coat the chicken with flour and dust off excess. Set aside. Heat 2 tbsp oil in a large skillet. Brown the chicken cutlets on both sides. Transfer to a plate. In the same skillet, add more olive oil if needed. Sauté mushrooms briefly on medium-high, about 1 minute or so. Then add tomatoes, garlic, the remaining ½ tbsp oregano, ½ tsp salt and ½ tsp pepper with 2 tsp flour. Cook for another 3 minutes or so, stirring regularly. Add wine, cook briefly to reduce a bit, then add lemon juice and broth. Bring to a boil then add chicken back to skillet. Cook over high for 3-4 minutes, then reduce heat to medium-low. Cover and cook for 8 minutes more until chicken is fully cooked. If you like, add a handful of baby spinach just before serving.

Easy Italian Baked Chicken

2 lb boneless free-range chicken breasts

Salt and pepper

2 tsp oregano

1 tsp fresh thyme

1 tsp paprika

4 garlic cloves, minced

3 tbsp extra virgin olive oil

Juice from 1 lemon

1 medium red onion, thinly sliced

5-6 small Roma tomatoes, halved

Preheat oven to 425°. Pat chicken dry. Place a breast in zip-top bag and close, pressing out air. Using a meat mallet, pound the chicken to flatten it. Repeat for all breasts. Season chicken with salt and pepper on both sides and set in a large bowl. Add spices, garlic, olive oil and lemon juice. Make sure chicken is evenly coated. In a large lightly oiled baking pan, spread onion slices on the bottom. Place chicken on top and then add tomatoes. Cover tightly with foil and bake for 10 minutes, then uncover and bake another 8-10 minutes. Remove from heat. Let chicken rest, covered, for 5-10 minutes more. Serve with fresh parsley or basil as garnish.

Sheet Pan Chicken Fajitas

1/3 cup olive oil

¼ cup freshly squeezed lime juice

2 tbsp fresh lime zest

1 tbsp honey

1 tsp cumin

1 tsp chili powder

1 tsp smoked paprika

½ tsp salt

½ tsp black pepper

2 garlic cloves, minced

2 bell peppers (red, orange or yellow)

1 sweet onion

1 lb free range chicken breasts, cut into 1" pieces

¼ cup chopped fresh cilantro, plus more for serving

Quick guacamole:

2 avocados

1-2 limes, juiced

2 tbsp diced onion

1 Roma tomato, diced

1/3 cup chopped cilantro

½ tsp cumin

Salt and pepper

. . .

Preheat oven to 425°. Spray a baking sheet with cooking spray. In a bowl, add the olive oil through garlic and whisk. Place the peppers and onions on the baking sheet. Add half the marinade and toss until well mixed. Roast in the oven for 15-20 minutes, tossing once or twice. In the meantime, place the chicken in a bowl and pour the remaining marinade over top. Let sit until vegetables are roasted. When vegetables are finished, toss them a few times and move them to one side of baking sheet. Place the chicken on baking sheet. Roast for 15 minutes or until done. Serve chicken and vegetables on gluten-free tortillas with guacamole and fresh cilantro.

Cilantro Lime Chicken

8 free-range chicken thighs

6 garlic cloves, chopped

1 cup dry white wine

2 limes, juiced

2 cups chicken broth

1 bunch cilantro, chopped

1 ½ tsp seasoned salt

1 tsp regular or hot paprika

1 tsp black pepper

1 tbsp garlic powder

½ tsp nutmeg

Preheat oven to 375°. In a small bowl, mix the spices. Pat the chicken dry and season pieces on both sides with spice mix. Let sit for 15 minutes. Heat 1-2 tbsp olive oil in cast iron (or oven proof) skillet. Brown chicken on both sides, then set aside. Lower the heat and deglaze the skillet with the wine. Let cook to reduce and then add broth. Bring to a simmer, then add lime juice and garlic. Return chicken to skillet and add cilantro. Bring to a simmer for 5 minutes. Cover and transfer to oven for 45 minutes or until chicken is cooked through. Remove from oven and let sit for 5 min, and then serve.

Garlic Rosemary Chicken with Cranberries

2 cups fresh cranberries

1/3 cup brown sugar

4 tbsp white wine vinegar

6 pieces bone-in free-range chicken

6-8 cloves garlic, minced

salt and pepper

1 ½ tbsp. chopped fresh (or 1 ½ tsp dried) rosemary

1 tsp paprika

1/3 cup extra virgin olive oil

1 lemon, juice of

1 large yellow onion, chopped

3 celery stalks, chopped

½ cup chicken broth

In a small bowl, combine cranberries, brown sugar and 2 tbsp of vinegar. Set aside. Pat the chicken dry. Rub with minced garlic on both sides, season with salt and pepper. Combine rosemary and paprika, then apply to chicken on both sides. In a large bowl, mix olive oil, lemon juice and remaining vinegar. Add the chicken, celery, onion and the used lemon halves. Mix and marinate for 15 minutes. Preheat oven to 425°. Heat 1 tbsp olive oil in skillet. Brown the chicken pieces on both sides. Place the chicken and used marinade in a lightly oiled baking pan. Add broth and the sugared cranberries. Bake for 35-40 minutes until chicken is cooked.

(Note: if using boneless chicken, bake time will be 25-30 minutes)

Cajun Shrimp

½ cup olive oil

2 tbsp parsley

2 tbsp Cajun/Creole seasoning

Juice of 1 lemon

2 tbsp honey

2 tbsp soy sauce (gluten-free)

1 lb wild caught shrimp, peeled and deveined

Mix all in a baking dish. Bake at 450° for 10-15 minutes, stirring occasionally. Serve over brown rice, cauliflower rice, or with gluten-free bread toasted.

Caribbean Shrimp

1 tbsp light brown sugar

1 tsp ground allspice

1 tsp black pepper

1 tsp onion powder

1 tsp garlic powder

1 tsp dried thyme

½ tsp salt

¼ tsp cayenne pepper

1 tbsp olive or grapeseed oil

1 tbsp molasses

2 tbsp fresh lime juice

1 ¾ cups jumbo wild caught shrimp, peeled and deveined

1 lime cut into wedges

Heat broiler. Coat broiler pan with non-stick cooking spray. Mix brown sugar through cayenne pepper in a bowl. Whisk in oil, molasses, and lime juice. Add shrimp and toss to coat. Cover and refrigerate 10 minutes, stirring after 5 minutes. Arrange shrimp in a single layer on broiler pan. Broil about 4" from heat for 2 minutes. Turn shrimp over. Broil 1-2 minutes or until shrimp are cooked through. Serve with rice.

Mediterranean Shrimp and Zucchini

1 ½ tbsp oregano

1 tsp cumin

1 tsp ground coriander

½ tsp paprika

1 lb large shrimp (wild caught), peeled and deveined

½ medium red onion, thinly sliced

5 garlic cloves, minced

1 bell pepper, sliced into sticks

1-2 zucchini, halved lengthwise then sliced

1 cup cooked chickpeas

1 ½ cups cherry tomatoes, halved

Salt and pepper

Juice from 1 large lemon

Fresh basil for garnish

Mix spices in a small bowl. Pat shrimp dry; season with sea salt and 1 ½ tsp of the spice mixture. Set aside. In a large skillet, heat 2 tbsp extra virgin olive oil over medium heat. Add onions and half the garlic and cook for 3-4 minutes. Add bell pepper, zucchini, and chickpeas. Season with salt and pepper and remaining spice mixture. Toss to combine. If needed, cook another 5 min or so until vegetables are tender. Transfer vegetables to a large plate. Add a little olive oil to skillet. Add the seasoned shrimp and remaining garlic. Cook over medium-high heat until shrimp are totally pink (about 4-5 minutes). Add the vegetables back to the skillet. Add tomatoes and lemon juice. Toss together, then serve with a garnish of fresh basil.

Mediterranean Baked Cod

1 ½ lb cod fillet pieces

5 garlic cloves, minced

½ cup chopped fresh parsley leaves

5 tbsp fresh lemon juice

5 tbsp extra virgin olive oil

2 tbsp melted organic butter

1/3 cup gluten-free flour (King Arthur Measure-for-Measure works best)

1 tsp ground coriander

¾ tsp smoked paprika

¾ tsp cumin

¾ tsp salt

½ tsp black pepper

Preheat oven to 400°. Mix lemon juice, olive oil and butter in a bowl; set aside. In another bowl, mix flour and spices. Set aside. Pat fish fillets dry. Dip fish in lemon juice mixture, then in flour mixture. Shake off extra flour. Heat 2 tbsp olive oil in skillet over medium-high heat. Add fish and sear on each side to give it some color, but do not fully cook (about a couple of minutes on each side). Remove from heat and place in baking pan. To the remaining lemon juice mixture, add the garlic and mix. Drizzle all over the fish fillets. Bake until fish begins to easily flake (about 10 minutes). Remove from heat and sprinkle fresh parsley on top and serve.

VEGAN

Portobello Burgers

4 portobello mushrooms, stemmed

1 tbsp olive oil

Salt and pepper

14 oz plum tomatoes

3 garlic cloves, sliced

¼ tsp red pepper flakes

Gluten-free buns, if desired

Line a baking sheet with parchment paper. Put mushrooms on baking sheet, stem side down. Brush with 1 ½ tsp oil and add salt and pepper. Toss tomatoes with remaining oil, garlic and red pepper flakes and add to mushrooms on baking sheet. Bake at 450°, flipping mushrooms and stirring tomatoes halfway through, for 25 minutes. Remove from oven and put the tomatoes in a bowl; set aside. Broil the buns, then broil mushrooms for 3 minutes. Flip and broil another 1-2 minutes.

Cuban Black Bean Stew

1 ½ cups brown rice

1 tbsp olive oil

1 medium red onion, chopped

1 garlic clove, minced

1 red pepper, chopped

2 cans organic black beans, rinsed and drained

14 oz vegetable broth

1 tbsp apple cider vinegar

½ tsp oregano

Salt and pepper

Lime and freshly chopped cilantro for garnish

Make rice. Sauté onion, garlic and red pepper in oil, about 8-10 minutes. Add beans through oregano. Cook another 6-8 minutes, mashing some of the beans to thicken. Season with salt and pepper to taste. Serve over brown rice with lime juice and cilantro as garnish.

Cilantro Lime Quinoa and Beans

1 cup quinoa

2 cups vegetable broth

2 tbsp lime juice

½ cup chopped fresh cilantro

1 can organic black beans, rinsed and drained

Salt and pepper to taste

Put quinoa and broth in saucepan and bring to a boil. Simmer for 15 minutes with lid on. Remove from heat for 5 minutes. Add rest, let sit 5 minutes to heat beans, then serve.

DESSERTS

Zucchini Brownies

1 cup creamy almond butter

1 egg

½ tsp sea salt

½ tsp baking powder

½ cup coconut sugar

½ tsp vanilla

½ cup dark chocolate chips

1 large zucchini, grated

Preheat oven to 350°. Line an 8x8" or similar size baking pan with parchment paper or spray with coconut baking spray. In large bowl, mix almond butter through vanilla. Fold in chocolate chips and zucchini. Spread evenly in pan. Bake for 25-30 minutes or until toothpick comes out clean.

Low Carb Brownie Batter Truffles

1 ¼ cup almond flour

Sugar substitute equivalent to ½ cup sugar

1/3 cup cocoa powder

Pinch of salt

½ cup butter, melted

1 tsp vanilla

3 oz sugar-free dark chocolate, chopped

1 tbsp coconut oil

Sprinkles (optional)

In a large bowl, whisk together the flour, sweetener, cocoa powder and salt. Stir in melted butter and vanilla until dough forms. If dough is too crumbly, add water 1 tbsp at a time until it sticks together. Freeze dough for 15 minutes. Roll into 1" balls and place on wax paper on baking sheet. Freeze at least 1 hour. In a double boiler or heatproof bowl over a simmering pan of water, mix chopped chocolate and coconut oil. Stir until melted and smooth. Drop a frozen truffle into the chocolate, tossing to coat thoroughly. Lift out with fork or small tongs and place back on baking sheet to set. If desired, add sprinkles for decoration now. Let harden.

Gluten-free, Dairy-free Pumpkin Pie

1 tsp coconut oil for pan

3 eggs

1/3 cup honey

15 oz can pumpkin

1 tbsp cinnamon

1 tbsp vanilla

2 tbsp coconut flour

1 cup unsweetened coconut milk

Grease a 9" pie pan with oil. Mix eggs through vanilla with a whisk. Sift flour in, and then add coconut milk. Bake at 350° for 75 minutes (cover edges at 45 min if browning). Cool for 2 hours on rack.

Chocolate Mint Dairy-Free Pudding

1 can coconut milk

2 tbsp vanilla

2 tbsp cocoa powder

Peppermint extract, to taste

Chill coconut milk in refrigerator for at least 15 minutes. Drain liquid from coconut milk, then put the solid component into a bowl. Add vanilla, cocoa powder and peppermint extract and mix. Refrigerate until ready to serve. Garnish with coconut, peppermint candy shavings, or dark chocolate chips.

FINAL THOUGHTS FROM AN
INTEGRATIVE PHYSICIAN

*N*ow that you know what toxins are out there and how important it is to maintain a clean lifestyle, you are equipped to achieve good health! Take your newfound knowledge and set goals. None of us (physicians included) eat perfectly and stay toxin-free all the time. In fact, I have a good friend who owns a winery. There are times when we get together that I will have an extra glass of her wonderful wine. Sometimes I just love bacon with my eggs on a Saturday morning. I have also indulged in too much dark chocolate when stressed or ice cream on a summer evening. But those things don't define my regular habits. When I was growing up, my parents called them "special treats". Walking to the ice cream store with Dad or having "sugar cereal" when we were camping were infrequent events indeed. When you indulge rarely, they will stay special treats and enhance life. Keep them special.

Working toward good health is a journey your holistic practitioner can help you with, but it is largely up to you. There is so much power in eating whole foods and maintaining good lifestyle habits. I often challenge my patients to get so healthy that they don't need me anymore and they put me out of business! I love helping people clean up their diet, sleep well, achieve a healthy weight and get off prescription medication.

 Our greatest happiness does not depend on the condition of life in which chance has placed us, but is always the result of a good conscience, good health, occupation, and freedom in all just pursuits.

— THOMAS JEFFERSON

Ask yourself: how healthy do I want to be ten years from now? Twenty years from now? Then ask yourself what you are willing to do get the results you want. Good health is a priceless treasure! Some of us seem to have it easily, but some of us have to work hard to achieve it. But along with faith, family, and love, health should be one of our highest priorities. I challenge you to invest time and effort into your health. I promise it's worth it!

REFERENCES

1. Centers for Disease Control and Prevention. *Fourth Rep ort on Human Exposure to Environmental Chemicals,* 2009. Atlanta, GA: U.S. Department of Health and Human Services, Centers for Disease Control and Prevention. https://www.cdc.gov/exposurereport/
2. Environmental Protection Agency, *Toxic Substances Control Act Chemical Substance Inventory,* https://www. epa.gov/tsca-inventory/how-access-tsca-inventory#download
3. Centers for Disease Control and Prevention. *Fourth Report on Human Exposure to Environmental Chemicals,* 2009. Atlanta, GA: U.S. Department of Health and Human Services, Centers for Disease Control and Prevention. https://www.cdc.gov/exposurereport/
4. Blount BC, et al. *Levels of seven urinary phthalate metabolites in a human reference population.* Environ Health Perspect. 2000; 108(10):979-82.
5. Calafat AM, et al. *Urinary concentrations of bisphenol A and 4-Nonylphenol in a human reference*

population. Environmental Health Perspectives. 2005; 113(4):391–395

6. Environmental Working Group, *A benchmark investigation of industrial chemicals, pollutants and pesticides in umbilical cord blood,* July 14, 2005

7. Seachrist DD et al. *A review of the carcinogenic potential of bisphenol A.* Reproductive Toxicology 2016. 59:167-182

8. .Shankar A, Teppala S. *Relationship between urinary bisphenol A levels and diabetes mellitus.* The Journal of Clinical Endocrinology & Metabolism. 2011;96:3822–3826.

9. Melzer D, et al. *Association of urinary bisphenol A concentration with heart disease: evidence from NHANES 2003/06,* PLOS One, published January 13, 2010

10. Carwile JL, Michels KB. *Urinary bisphenol A and obesity: NHANES 2003–2006.* Environmental Research. 2011;111(6):825–830

11. Benjamin, S. *Phthalates impact human health: Epidemiological evidences and plausible mechanism of action,* J Hazard Mater, 2017 Oct 15;340:360-383.

12. Fisher, J. *Environmental anti-androgens and male reproductive health: focus on phthalates and testicular dysgenesis syndrome,* Reproduction 2004: 127(3):305-315

13. Wenzel, A. et al. *Prevalence and predictors of phthalate exposure in pregnant women in Charleston, SC,* Chemosphere 2018;193:394-402.

14. Boberg, J. et al. *Possible endocrine disrupting effects of parabens and their metabolites.* Reproductive Toxicology 2010 Sept 30(2):301-12

15. Gorini, F. *The Role of Polybrominated Diphenyl Ethers in Thyroid Carcinogenesis: Is It a Weak Hypothesis or a Hidden Reality? From Facts to New Perspectives.* Int J Environ Res Public Health. 2018 Sep; 15(9):1834.

16. National Institute Of Environmental Health Sciences.

Certain PCBs Linked To Increased Risk Of Cancer. Science Daily, 10 November 2004.

17. Raffetti E, Donato F, De Palma G, Leonardi L, Sileo C, Magoni M. *Polychlorinated biphenyls (PCBs) and risk of dementia and Parkinson disease: A population-based cohort study in a North Italian highly polluted area.* Chemosphere. 2020 Dec;261:127522.

18. Goldman, S. et al., *Polychlorinated biphenyls (PCBs) and Parkinson's disease (PD): effect modification by membrane transporter variants (S32.004),* Neurology, Apr 2016, 86 (16 Supplement)

19. Lilis, R., et al. *Prevalence of disease among vinyl chloride and polyvinyl chloride workers.* Annals of the New York Academy of Sciences, 1975. 246: 22-41

20. Hayes, T. et al. *Demasculinization and feminization of male gonads by atrazine: consistent effects across vertebrate classes,* The Journal of Steroid Biochemistry and Molecular Biology, Volume 127, Issues 1–2, 2011, pages 64-73.

21. Donna, A. et al. *Triazine herbicides and ovarian epithelial neoplasms.* Scand. J. Work Environ. Health, 15: 47(1989).

22. Yueh, MF et al. *Triclosan promotes liver fibrosis and tumor growth.* Proceedings of the National Academy of Sciences Dec 2014, 111 (48) 17200-17205.

23. Crofton KM, Paul KB, Devito MJ, Hedge JM. *Short-term in vivo exposure to the water contaminant triclosan: evidence for disruption of thyroxine.* Environ Toxicol Pharmacol. 2007 Sep;24(2):194-7.

24. Bertelsen RJ, et al. *Triclosan exposure and allergic sensitization in Norwegian children.* Allergy. 2013 Jan;68(1):84-91.

25. Sagiv SK, et al. *Prenatal organophosphate pesticide exposure and traits related to autism spectrum disorders in a population living in proximity to agriculture.* Environ Health Perspect. 2018 Apr 25;126(4):047012

26. Eskenazi, B., et al. *Association of in utero organophosphate pesticide exposure and fetal growth and length of gestation in an agricultural population.* Environ Health Perspect. 2004 Jul;112(10):1116-24

27. Eskenazi, B., et al. *Exposures of children to organophosphate pesticides and their potential adverse health effects.* Environ Health Perspect. 107:409-419.

28. Raanan R, Harley KG, Balmes JR, Bradman A, Lipsett M, Eskenazi B. *Early-life exposure to organophosphate pesticides and pediatric respiratory symptoms in the CHAMACOS cohort. Environ Health Perspect.* 2015;123(2):179-185.

29. https://www.npr.org/2020/06/24/882949098/bayer-to-pay-more-than-10-billion-to-resolve-roundup-cancer-lawsuits

30. Clair, E., et al. *A glyphosate-based herbicide induces necrosis and apoptosis in mature rat testicular cells in vitro, and testosterone decrease at lower levels,* Toxicology in Vitro, Volume 26, Issue 2, 2012, Pages 269-279.

31. Paola Ingaramo, Ramiro Alarcón, Mónica Muñoz-de-Toro, Enrique H. Luque, *Are glyphosate and glyphosate-based herbicides endocrine disruptors that alter female fertility?,* Molecular and Cellular Endocrinology, 2020. Volume 518, 110934.

32. Samsel, A., Seneff, S. *Glyphosate's suppression of cytochrome P450 enzymes and amino acid biosynthesis by the gut microbiome: pathways to modern diseases,* 2013. Entropy 15, 1416-1463.

33. https://archive.epa.gov/mtbe/web/html/water.html

34. https://www.atsdr.cdc.gov/phs/phs.asp?id=226&tid=41

35. McGwin G, Lienert J, Kennedy JI. *Formaldehyde exposure and asthma in children: a systematic review.* Environ Health Perspect. 2010 Mar;118(3):313-7.

36. https://www.epa.gov/indoor-air-quality-iaq/volatile-organic-compounds-impact-indoor-air-quality

37. https://cfpub.epa.gov/ncea/iris/iris_documents/documents/subst/0106_summary.pdf

38. https://www.epa.gov/sites/production/files/2016-09/documents/xylenes.pdf

39. Nissen MS, et al. *Sinonasal adenocarcinoma following styrene exposure in the reinforced plastics industry.* Occup Environ Med. 2018 Jun;75(6):412-414.

40. Christensen, M., et al. *Styrene exposure and risk of lymphohematopoietic malignancies in 73,036 reinforced plastics workers,* Epidemiology: May 2018; 29(3):342-351.

41. https://www.epa.gov/sites/production/files/2016-05/documents/pfoa_hesd_final_508.pdf

42. Smith MT. *Advances in understanding benzene health effects and susceptibility.* Annu Rev Public Health. 2010;31:133-148.

43. Rice JM. *The carcinogenicity of acrylamide.* Mutat Res. 2005 Feb 7;580(1-2):3-20.

44. https://www.atsdr.cdc.gov/phs/phs.asp?id=1113&tid=236

45. Somers EC, et al. *Mercury exposure and antinuclear antibodies among females of reproductive age in the United States: NHANES.* Environ Health Perspect; [Online 10 February 2015].

46. Langford N, Ferner R. *Toxicity of mercury.* J Hum Hypertens. 1999 Oct;13(10):651-6.

47. Oberoi S, Barchowsky A, Wu F. *The global burden of disease for skin, lung, and bladder cancer caused by arsenic in food.* Cancer Epidemiol Biomarkers Prev. 2014 Jul;23(7):1187-94.

48. Delgado CF, et al. *Lead exposure and developmental disabilities in preschool-aged children.* J Public Health Manag Pract. 2018 Mar/Apr;24(2):e10-e17.

49. Johri N, Jacquillet G, Unwin R. *Heavy metal poisoning: the*

effects of cadmium on the kidney. Biometals. 2010
Oct;23(5):783-92.

50. Alfvén T, et al. *Low-level cadmium exposure and osteoporosis.*
J Bone Miner Res. 2000 Aug;15(8):1579-86.

51. Conklin DJ, et al. *Biomarkers of chronic acrolein inhalation
exposure in mice: implications for tobacco product-induced
toxicity.* Toxicol Sci. 2017 Aug 1;158(2):263-274

52. Steinmaus CM. *Perchlorate in water supplies: sources,
exposures, and health effects.* Curr Environ Health Rep.
2016 Jun;3(2):136-43.

53. https://www.cdc.gov/tobacco/campaign/tips/
diseases/cancer.html

54. Paterni I, Granchi C, Minutolo F. *Risks and benefits related
to alimentary exposure to xenoestrogens.* Crit Rev Food Sci
Nutr. 2017 Nov 2;57(16):3384-3404.

55. Roomruangwong C, Carvalho AF, Comhaire F, Maes M.
*Lowered plasma steady-state levels of progesterone combined
with declining progesterone levels during the luteal phase
predict peri-menstrual syndrome and its major subdomains.*
Front Psychol. 2019 Oct 30;10:2446.

56. Sarmah S, Muralidharan P, Marrs JA. *Common congenital
anomalies: Environmental causes and prevention with folic
acid containing multivitamins.* Birth Defects Res C Embryo
Today. 2016 Sep;108(3):274-286.

57. Mima M, Greenwald D, Ohlander S. *Environmental toxins
and male fertility.* Curr Urol Rep. 2018 May 17;19(7):50.

58. Pizzorno J. *Environmental toxins and infertility.* Integr Med
(Encinitas). 2018 Apr;17(2):8-11.

59. Shankar A, Teppala S. *Relationship between urinary
bisphenol A levels and diabetes mellitus.* The Journal of
Clinical Endocrinology &
Metabolism. 2011;96:3822–3826.

60. Benjamin, S. *Phthalates impact human health:*

Epidemiological evidences and plausible mechanism of action, J Hazard Mater, 2017 Oct 15;340:360-383.

61. https://ndnr.com/autoimmuneallergy-medicine/how-environmental-toxicants-contribute-to-allergy-asthma-and-autoimmunity/

62. Modabbernia A, Velthorst E, Reichenberg A. *Environmental risk factors for autism: an evidence-based review of systematic reviews and meta-analyses.* Mol Autism. 2017 Mar 17;8:13.

63. Curtis LT, Patel K. *Nutritional and environmental approaches to preventing and treating autism and attention deficit hyperactivity disorder (ADHD): a review.* J Altern Complement Med. 2008 Jan-Feb;14(1):79-85.

64. Rzhetsky A, Bagley SC, Wang K, Lyttle CS, Cook EH Jr, et al. *Environmental and state-level regulatory factors affect the incidence of autism and intellectual disability.* PLOS Computational Biology 2014 Mar 13;10(3)

65. Dickerson AS, Rahbar MH, Han I, et al. *Autism spectrum disorder prevalence and proximity to industrial facilities releasing arsenic, lead or mercury.* Sci Total Environ 2015;536:245-251.

66. Hales CM, Carroll MD, Fryar CD, Ogden CL. *Prevalence of obesity and severe obesity among adults: United States, 2017–2018.* NCHS Data Brief, no 360. Hyattsville, MD: National Center for Health Statistics. 2020

67. Silva V, et al, *Distribution of glyphosate and aminomethylphosphonic acid (AMPA) in agricultural topsoils of the European Union,* Science of The Total Environment, Volume 621, 2018, Pages 1352-1359.

68. Jackson E, Shoemaker R, Larian N, Cassis, L. *Adipose tissue as a site of toxin accumulation.* Compr Physiol 2017 Sep 12;7(4):1085-1135.

69. Roszkowska A, Pawlicka M, Mroczek A, Bałabuszek K,

Nieradko-Iwanicka B. *Non-celiac gluten sensitivity: a review.* Medicina (Kaunas). 2019 May 28;55(6):222.

70. Benbrook, C.M. *Trends in glyphosate herbicide use in the United States and globally. Environ* Sci Eur 28, 3 (2016).

71. Storhaug, C. et al. *Country, regional, and global estimates for lactose malabsorption in adults: a systemic review and meta-analysis.* The Lancet Gastroenterology and Hepatology 2017, 2(10): 738-746.

72. https://www.ewg.org/foodnews/summary.php#.Wrlu9pPwbGI

73. Bradman A, et al. *Effect of organic diet intervention on pesticide exposures in young children living in low-income urban and agricultural communities.* Environ Health Perspect. 2015 Oct;123(10):1086-93.

74. https://www.cancer.gov/about-cancer/causes-prevention/risk/diet/cooked-meats-fact-sheet

75. Di Minno MN, Franchini M, Russolillo A, Lupoli R, Iervolino S, Di Minno G. *Alcohol dosing and the heart: updating clinical evidence.* Semin Thromb Hemost. 2011 Nov;37(8):875-84

76. Grewal P, Viswanathen VA. *Liver cancer and alcohol.* Clin Liver Dis. 2012 Nov;16(4):839-50.

77. Saluk-Juszczak J, Wachowicz B. *Aktywność prozapalna lipopolisacharydu [The proinflammatory activity of lipopolysaccharide].* Postepy Biochem. 2005;51(3):280-7.

78. Krause AJ, Simon EB, Mander BA, et al. *The sleep-deprived human brain.* Nat Rev Neurosci. 2017;18(7):404-418.

79. Tomasi D, et al. *Impairment of attentional networks after 1 night of sleep deprivation.* Cereb Cortex. 2009 Jan;19(1):233-40.

80. Rasmussen MK, Mestre H, Nedergaard M. *The glymphatic pathway in neurological disorders.* Lancet Neurol. 2018 Nov;17(11):1016-1024.

81. Watson NF, Badr MS, Belenky G, et al. *Recommended*

Amount of Sleep for a Healthy Adult: A Joint Consensus Statement of the American Academy of Sleep Medicine and Sleep Research Society. Sleep. 2015;38(6):843-844.

82. Fietze I, et al. *Prevalence and association analysis of obstructive sleep apnea with gender and age differences - Results of SHIP-Trend.* J Sleep Res. 2019 Oct;28(5):e12770.

ABOUT THE AUTHOR

Gretchen Reis, MD is board certified in both Family Medicine and Integrative Medicine and specializes in bioidentical hormone therapy and anti-aging medicine. She is passionate about combining nutrition, healthy lifestyle habits, bioidentical hormones and nutritional supplements to help her patients achieve optimal health.

She graduated from Baylor College of Medicine in Houston, Texas, and then completed a residency in Family Medicine in Lancaster, Pennsylvania. She practiced family medicine in Pennsylvania for several years before moving to Ohio, where she had a rural solo family medicine practice for 10 years.

Fascinated with a natural approach to medicine, she transitioned to Integrative Medicine with an emphasis on bioidentical hormone therapy. She started her anti-aging practice in Charlotte, North Carolina in 2013.

She and her staff at Integrity Wellness MD offer bioidentical hormone therapy, aesthetic treatments, weight loss, and integrative medicine. She is a member of the North Carolina Integrative Medical Society and the American Academy of Anti-Aging Medicine.

She and her husband live just across the border in South Carolina with the youngest two of their four adopted children.

CPSIA information can be obtained
at www.ICGtesting.com
Printed in the USA
BVHW062337010321
601388BV00009B/918

9 781736 313909